Yoga Guide for Beginners

101 Poses and Sequences for Strength, Flexibility, and Mindfulness

Contents

About Yoga

What is Yoga

Hello and welcome! This book is targeted at beginner yoga practitioners. They're known as *yogis* (from the Classical Sanskrit word *yogin*). A yogi can be male or female. The term for a female yoga practitioner is *yogini,* but it is not widely used.

Broadly speaking, yoga refers to a collection of practices for body, mind, and soul which originated in ancient India. Etymologically, *yoga* stems from the Sanskrit root *yuj* which means "to add" or "to unite."

Essentially, yoga is more than physical exercise. It is a meditative practice with a spiritual core. Through its practice, yogis seek to reach the *moksha*, "liberation." This liberation refers to "breaking out" of the cycle of death and rebirth. It means liberating ourselves from ignorance.

The precise definition of the term "yoga" varies with the context, but most of the time it refers to:

- A disciplined method of achieving a goal
- A set of techniques to control both mind and body
- A school of philosophy
- In conjunction with other prefixes, a traditional set of techniques and philosophies (yoga schools)
- The practice of yoga

Yoga involves static principles that vary *slightly* from one school to another while maintaining the same ultimate purpose: the liberation.

This refers to yoga as a means of discovering the dysfunctions in our perception and cognition. Through yoga, we overcome these to *liberate* ourselves from suffering, bringing forth inner peace and salvation.

By meditating with yoga, we raise and expand our consciousness. We change the lens to become coextensively aware with all that surrounds us and not just ourselves.

Yogis *must* carve a path to omniscience and heightened consciousness with yoga. The end goal is breaking our chains to falsehood and suffering. We are meant to understand both the impermanent and permanent realities that clash in life.

Please note that in case you are pregnant, nursing, have sustained injuries or have any other condition that might conflict with you practicing yoga, it's important to consult the appropriate health services first before starting with yoga.

About Yoga Schools and Hatha Yoga

It is important to understand that *all* yoga schools stem from "classical yoga", which is considered one of the *āstika* (Sanskrit word for "there it is" or "exists") schools of Hinduism.

In effect, yoga refers to a variety of schools with their own practices, methods, and philosophies extending to different Jain, Buddhist, and Hindu practices.

Amongst these Hindu schools, we can find Jnana yoga, Karma yoga, Bhakti yoga, and Hatha yoga, among others.

Hatha yoga ("Hatha" being the Sanskrit word for "force") focuses on exercises to cultivate strength both physical and mental. The exercises in question are none other than the poses adopted in yoga, called *asanas* (the Sanskrit word for "sitting down" or "to sit down").

For this reason, this book will focus on Hatha yoga. While other yoga schools *do* have the asanas as well, Hatha yoga is *focused* on mastering the body through them.

Hatha yoga is about using diet to purify our body, *pranayama* (breathing techniques) to master our life energy, and the asanas to master our physical abilities, obtaining the *siddhis* (special body powers) in the process.

Traditionally speaking, there are a few rules for performing the asanas:

- Asanas *should* be performed while fasting.
- Force *should not* be applied. The body *should not* tremble.
- The parts of the body *should* be moved slowly, particularly the head and heels.

- The breathing *should* be controlled (referred to as "*pranayama*", the Sanskrit word for "breath control" or "control of the breath"; more about it later).
- Stress from the body *should* be released with special poses *before* performing other asanas.

Following these traditional rules, while not mandatory, can be very helpful for any prospective yogi.

It would be wise to remember that practicing yoga should be comfortable regardless of your skill level. You shouldn't push your body into discomfort at any point. Try your best *not to* turn yoga into a competition with yourself.

The goal here is mastering your body. Beginners won't feel too comfortable at the start; it will take several short sessions with relatively simple poses. As the yogi advances, he or she becomes unattached from the feeling of discomfort.

This is vital to reach the spiritual goal of yoga, which is detachment from suffering.

Besides the asanas, Hatha yoga extends to other practices. The philosophy behind it states that a successful yogi should display the following characteristics:

- *Utsaha* ("enthusiasm" or "fortitude")
- *Sahasa* ("courage" or "optimism")
- *Dhairya* ("patience" or "persistence")
- *Jnana Tattva* ("knowledge")
- *Nishcaya* ("resolve" or "determination")
- *Tyaga* ("solitude" or "renunciation")

It's easy for westerners to assume that Hatha yoga (or even yoga in general) is *exclusively* about the asanas.

Despite this mistaken conception, Hatha yoga encompasses more than that. It blends different ideas such as ethics, diet, cleansing, breathing and physical exercises, meditation, and spiritual development.

Consequently, to be a proper yogi one should reflect on the following practices:

✓ **"Proper" Diet**

Special emphasis is given to *mitahara* (the Sanskrit word that translates to "habit of moderate food"). It consists of a heightened awareness about food, drink, diet, and consumption habits.

Ancient texts refer to *mitahara* as a concept that links proper nutrition with the health of the body and mind. Some of the largest nutrition compendiums that have survived from ancient India highlight the importance of planning a diet.

The *Charaka Samhita* ("Compendium of Charaka") states that "wholesome diets promote health and growth." This concept, while coming from a collection of books that date from the pre-2nd century CE, is in perfect accord with modern thinking.

The general idea of *mitahara* is that we should tailor our diet according to our body, health, climate, season, habits, and tastes as well as constantly rotating what we eat to avoid excesses.

✓ **Proper "body cleansing"**

This refers to a series of practices to cleanse the body with the help of a yoga teacher.
These are beyond the scope of this book. However, I will briefly list them here in case you are curious:

➤ Netī

Yogic system for the cleaning of our air passageways. In simpler words, nasal wash with purified water and non-iodized salt.

This practice is wonderful for those who suffer nasal problems, but it should be performed with the aid of an expert and only after proper medical examination.

➤ Dhautī

Yogic system of body cleansing techniques. This practice is directed to the cleaning of the digestive and respiratory tracts, and the external ears and eyes.

➢ Naulī

Yogic system for cleaning the digestive organs. It is based on massage of the internal belly organs.

➢ Basti

Yogic system for the cleaning of the lower abdomen. These techniques involve delicate methods and should only be practiced with the help of experts.

➢ Kapālabhātī

Yogic system for "skull polishing". In other words, a set of practices to energize the brain.

➢ Trāṭaka

Yogic meditation method. It consists in staring at a single point (generally a candle flame) for a period of time to "bring energy to the third eye" and to enhance our ability to concentrate.

Its purpose is to give a rest to our minds. Thus we're "cleaning" our thoughts.

✓ **"Proper" breathing**

As mentioned before, "breath control" or pranayama refers to achieving the proper way of breathing through a set of techniques to alter how we breathe.

The intention is to produce specific positive results to amplify our life force.

Several forms of pranayama exist, and they're often based on *puraka* (inhalation), *kumbhaka* (retention), and *recaka* (exhalation). Each element can get very complex, but the general idea should be enough for starters.

The Origins of Yoga

It is said that yoga originated in pre-Vedic (3300 BCE) India, as some Indus Valley seals depict human figures performing what look like common yoga or meditation poses such as the headstand. However, these interpretations are considered uncertain and inconclusive.

Traditional Hinduism regards the Vedas (a large body of knowledge texts from ancient India) as the ultimate source of spiritual knowledge. These texts describe several ascetic practices (which include meditation and the use of bodily poses), and many scholars believe that they *might* have been precursors to yoga.

The characteristic elements of yoga were practiced, but no direct evidence of it being "yoga" exists.

Textual reference to yoga began to emerge in texts dating from 500–200 BCE. The first appearance of the term with the same meaning is found in the *Katha Upanishad*. The scriptures define yoga as "the steady control of the senses." Along with conscious control of our mental activity, it leads to a supreme state.

This connects with the modern definition of yoga as a process of interiorization and ascension.

The classical era (200 BCE–500 CE) saw many texts that systematically compiled several methods and practices for yoga.

Hatha yoga specifically surfaced during the Middle Ages (500–1500 CE). This period displayed several improvements and refinements to the traditions of yoga.

One of the first references to Hatha yoga can be found in Buddhist texts from the 8th century. However, the earliest full definition is found in the 11th-century Buddhist text *Vimalaprabha*. It refined the bodily poses (asanas) into the full range of body poses that are popular today.

The 15th century CE saw the birth of the Hathapradīpika, one of the most influential compilations of Hatha yoga. It included information about the six acts of body cleansing, the asanas, pranayama, meditation and other topics.

Thanks to the open nature of Hatha yoga, which did not limit its practices to persons of a specific sex, caste, class or creed, it quickly became a broader movement. A word about the traditional goal of Hatha yoga. The original objective of Hatha yoga was to attain physical *siddhis* (read as special powers or characteristics such as slowed aging) as well as "liberation" (*moksha*). These *siddhis* are more symbolic than anything else, merely a reflection of the soteriological desires of Indian religions.

Health Benefits of Yoga

Yoga offers several benefits to perseverant yogis.

Constant physical exercise, coupled with strong meditation and focus, leads to better health and well-being. This extends to the mind and the body.

It is important that you never forget that yoga is about transcendence. A prospective yogi should seek to strengthen his body, mind, and soul. This will lead him into a path of tranquility and peace.

Let's break down the many benefits of yoga into physical and mental categories.

Physical Benefits

Yoga *is not* an aerobic exercise (except some of the most complex poses). However, constant (as in daily) yoga exercise *will* help you build up muscle and burn calories.

For those who suffer from diabetes or other insulin-related problems, yoga allows your body to re-oxygenate at a better rate, breathing more life into your cells. In turn, this helps you regulate your blood sugar level.

Yoga poses stimulate your lymphatic system. This boosts your immune system and releases toxins from your body. Those who start practicing yoga regularly often experience a surge of energy. This can be attributed to the fact that oxygenated blood allows our bodies to perform much better.

Yoga exercise, along with controlled breathing and thoughtful meditation, can increase your overall energy. Lack of sleep, sedentary habits, and piled up stress can lead us to feel like we're at half our potential all the time. Yoga lets you recover from that!

Yogis who practice constantly reach a point at which they can push their physical boundaries far beyond what they could initially. This leads to better physical balance and more agility.

So, in a nutshell, practicing yoga will grant your body the following benefits:

- ✓ Increased flexibility and agility
- ✓ Stronger and better toned muscles
- ✓ More energy and vitality
- ✓ Improved respiration and metabolism
- ✓ Reduced weight (closer to your ideal weight)
- ✓ Better cardiovascular and circulatory health
- ✓ Higher athletic performance

Mental Benefits

Our everyday life is full of countless stressors that make *everything* harder. As it piles on, stress takes a whole new toll on our bodies because it triggers the release of cortisol and adrenaline (also known as the "survival" hormones).

I'm sure that you've felt a sudden rush of energy and hastiness after a heated argument or before an important event. That's stress for you!

The surplus of "survival hormones" in our bodies serves a purpose in real survival situations, but not in our everyday life. Many of us have a hard time managing our stress levels.

Fortunately, yoga is one of the many beneficial practices that help you relax your body. With constant practice, we learn how to release muscle tension on demand, and when we get our needed dose of stretching and breathing our body responds by triggering the release of certain "relaxation" hormones like serotonin.

20-minute yoga sessions inject more oxygen into our bloodstream, and that blood gets carried into our brain.

As we lower our stress levels, our immune system is strengthened. On the other hand, high levels of cortisol in our blood lead to a depressed immune system.

All in all, this leads to improvements in our quality of life. Better sleep is often a result of daily yoga practice.

The best part is that the mental benefits of yoga function pretty much like a positive feedback cycle. You sleep better, then you have less stress, then you have a better outlook on life—which in turn makes you sleep better!

The benefits of yoga are plentiful. You won't be lifting weights or running, but you will be cultivating your inner balance.

Some people dismiss these concepts, but the truth is that sometimes we need to take a moment to think about ourselves.

That is the primordial offer of yoga: thoughtful meditation and self-reconnection tied together with a series of poses to stretch our bodies.

So, in a nutshell, practicing yoga will grant your mind the following benefits:

- ✓ Increased focus
- ✓ Reduced stress levels
- ✓ Diminished anxiety and fidgetiness
- ✓ More motivation and willpower
- ✓ More happiness
- ✓ Heightened empathy
- ✓ Increased emotional resilience

About Pranayama

The breathing techniques of pranayama are vital for yoga, as there's an underlying link between the asanas and pranayama.

You see, in a conventional yoga class, with a yoga teacher, you're taught to *consciously* control your breathing. Many of us are accustomed to *just* breathing, period.

We don't inhale or exhale because we want to; it's just autopilot.

When practicing yoga, the efficiency of both your physical exercise and spiritual meditation can be measured by your breathing.

Breathing consciously allows you to maintain balance, it gives you more strength, endurance, and flexibility, and above everything it gives you peace to reconnect with your inner self.

Learn the following techniques, and try to add them during your asanas.

> **Ocean Breath (in Sanskrit "*Ujjayi Pranayama*")**

This is a classic breathing technique, perfect for relaxation and meditation.

To perform it during your yoga practice: Focus solely on your breath, inhaling deeply through your nose and then exhaling slowly, audibly making the "ah" sound. Repeat a couple of times, and then close your mouth.

> **Alternating Nostril Breath (in Sanskrit "*Nadi Shodhana Pranayama*")**

This therapeutic breathing technique allows you to clean and unblock your nasal cavities.

To perform it during your yoga practice: Finish your asana sequence, and then prepare your mind to meditate or relax.

Bring your right hand in front of your nose, close your right nostril with your thumb, and inhale through the left nostril. Now close your left nostril with your right forefinger, open the right nostril, and exhale slowly through it. Now switch (inhale through the right nostril and exhale through the left) and complete the cycle. Repeat it from 3 to 5 times.

> ### Breath Retention (in Sanskrit *"Kumbhaka Pranayama"*)

This breathing technique lets you improve your lung capacity.

To perform it during your asana practice: Finish your asana sequence, and then prepare your mind to meditate or relax.

Inhale as much as you can, filling your lungs to the max. Hold your breath for 10 seconds, and then try to inhale even more. Exhale, and wait a few seconds before trying it again. Do it 3 to 5 times.

> ### Breath of Fire (in Sanskrit *"Kapalabhati Pranayama"*)

This rapid breathing technique is meant to give you a kick-start when you're feeling lethargic or mentally numb.

To perform it during your asana practice: Take a deep inhale, and then exhale slowly. Now, inhale again, deeply, but exhale quickly, using your lower abs to push the air out. The trick is inhaling slowly and deeply, and then exhaling quickly. Repeat this process between 25 and 30 times.

> ### Short Breathing Tips

Generally, you should:

- **Exhale when bending forward.**
- **Inhale when lifting or puffing the chest.**
- **Exhale as you twist.**

101 Yoga Poses

The bread and butter of modern yoga: The asanas!

This book contains 101 different yoga poses that you can mix and match to design your own sequences. The poses have been ordered in their category from easiest to the hardest. The poses have also been divided in different categories to match where their main focus is. These include warm-up, neck, arms, wrists & shoulders, chest, hips, back, legs, and whole body. Nonetheless, several poses could have been included in several categories, so it's a good idea to look at the focus of each poses.

Each pose includes its focus, the physical indications and contraindications, time to hold the pose, its Sanskrit name, and the level aimed (beginner, intermediate, or advanced).

I suggest you plan your sessions so that every two days you switch your focus. For example, Monday and Tuesday you work on stretching your legs, and Wednesday and Thursday you work on stretching your arms.

Following the 101 poses, you will find 10 sequences you can use for different situations and that are ideal for the beginner yogi.

General tips

➢ Once you're done with a pose, don't rush to the next one! Transition to your new pose with calm and grace. It is important that you invite harmony and peace to yourself when practicing yoga.

➢ Don't force yourself to perform complex poses. Some people have the mistaken assumption that they can go straight for the Firefly (*Tittibhasana*) pose just because they go to the gym every day. That is not the case! Yoga is a different beast altogether, and you need to go steady and slow.

➢ Don't do over 40 minutes. As you acquire more skill, you'll be met with uncomfortable poses that will require many weeks of practice to pull off. 20 to 40-minute sessions are your best bet (I prefer the 20-minute ones). I'm referring here to the actual physical exercise. Typical yoga classes last about an hour, but they include a meditation and warm-up section. Don't extend your asana practice beyond 40 minutes.

➤ Count with breaths. Each pose should be held for as long as 3 to 5 deep, controlled breaths. First you must inhale slowly, then you must hold the air, then you exhale slowly. Be sure to work on the consistency of each breath!

➤ Don't mix more than 20 poses. You might be eager to try a lot of poses in a single day, but generally, doing 10 to 15 a day is more than enough. If you really want to push it, 20 should be your max. Constantly practicing, improving, and lastly, mastering, poses is far better for you.

➤ If a pose involves one side of your body, then it must be mirrored on the other side as well. So, if you stretch to the left for 3 breaths, you must stretch to the right for 3 breaths too.

Yoga Poses for Warming-Up

Mountain Pose

Focus: Thighs; knees; ankles; abdomen
Level: Beginner
Sanskrit Name: *Tadasana*
Time: At least a minute
Indications: Strengthening; stretching; improves pose
Contraindications: Headache; insomnia; low blood pressure

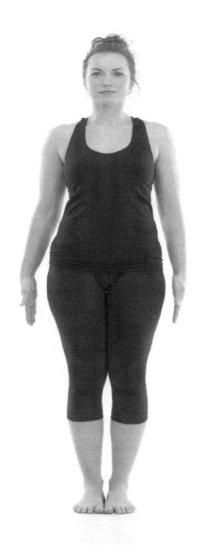

The Mountain Pose is the quintessential pose from which most standing poses begin. It improves your alignment; strengthens your thighs, knees, and ankles; and firms your torso and buttocks.

It's a great pose to follow up (or prepare for) the Downward Facing Dog Pose, and it can be used before or after most standing poses.

To perform this exercise, you must:

1. Stand firmly, with the bases of your big toes touching. Your heels should be slightly apart, so that your second toes are parallel.
2. Lift the toes and balls of your feet, spreading them thoroughly as you lay them gently on the floor. Move them back and forth and side to side. Gradually come to a stop, balancing your weight evenly on your feet.
3. Firm your thigh muscles and raise your kneecaps. Don't harden your lower belly.
4. Lift your inner ankles to strengthen the arches, then turn your upper thighs slightly inward.
5. Lengthen your tailbone toward the floor and then move your pubis toward your navel.
6. Send your shoulder blades into your back, and then widen them and press them down into your back. Lift the top of your sternum toward the ceiling without pushing your ribs forward.
7. Widen your collarbones and then hang your arms along your torso.
8. Balance the crown of your head over the center of your pelvis, keeping your chin parallel to the floor.
9. Hold the pose for a minute.

As you become more skilled, try doing this pose with your eyes closed, while breathing easily and evenly. This will help you attain inner balance.

Three even breaths should be long enough for this pose.

Staff Pose

Focus: Back; shoulders; chest
Level: Beginner
Sanskrit Name: *Dandasana*
Time: At least a minute
Indications: Stretching; strengthening; improves pose
Contraindications: Back injuries; wrist injuries

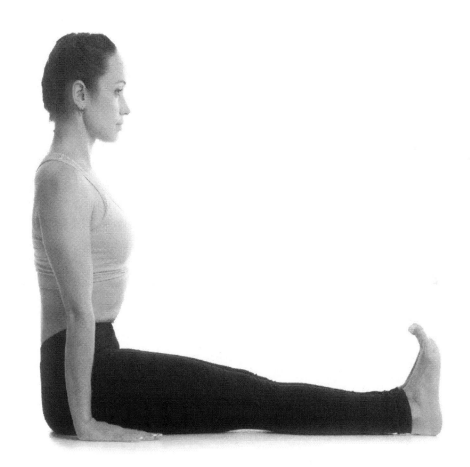

The Staff Pose is a straightforward seated pose to strengthen the back, shoulders and chest. It helps those with poor pose habits to adopt a correct pose.

To perform this exercise, you must:

1. Sit on the floor with your legs together and extended. If you feel like you can't keep your hamstrings from dragging your torso, you might want to lift your pelvis with a blanket or a bolster.
2. Adjust your pubis and tailbone to be equidistant from the floor.
3. Firm your thighs, press them against the floor, and then rotate them slightly to face each other.
4. Draw your inner groins towards the sacrum.
5. Flex your ankles and firmly press your palms against the floor.

If you're not sure about your alignment, try doing the exercise leaning against a wall. If your alignment is correct, your sacrum and shoulder blades *should* touch the wall. Your lower back and head *shouldn't*. You might want to put a small soft object, such as a rolled-up towel or cloth, between your lower back and the wall.

Laying some heavy objects (such as sandbags) on top of your thighs will help you ground them.

This seemingly-simple pose has more than meets the eye. You should imagine your spine as a staff, rooted firmly in the ground. Hold the pose for 3 to 5 even breaths. I recommend spending *at least* a whole minute like this.

Easy Pose

Focus: Knees; ankles; back
Level: Beginner
Sanskrit Name: *Sukhasana*
Time: At least 3 minutes
Indications: Stretching; strengthening; mental relaxation
Contraindications: Knee injuries

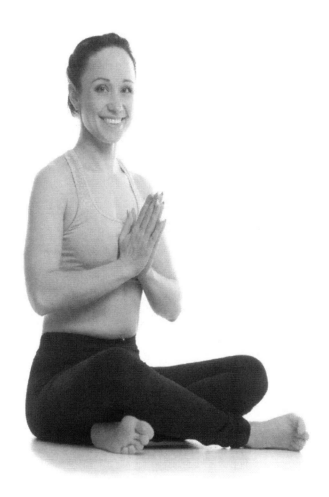

The Easy Pose is a seemingly simple pose that will challenge beginners accustomed to working long hours while sitting.

It stimulates the brain; lets you meditate; strengthens the back; and stretches knees and ankles.

I suggest sliding a folded blanket or two in the area you're going to practice; this will be your support.

To perform this exercise, you must:

1. Sit close to the edge of your blanket support, and then extend your legs out in front of you, as if you were performing the Staff Pose.
2. Cross your shins while you widen your legs, and then slip each foot beneath the opposite knee as you bend your knees and fold your legs toward your torso.
3. Be sure to keep your feet relaxed so that the outer edges rest on the floor while the inner arches settle below the opposite shin. Ideally, you should discern a triangle between your two thighs and crossed shins. The gap between feet and pelvis should be comfortable, not closed.
4. Sit with your pelvis relatively neutral. To achieve this, press your hands against your blanket support, make your thigh bones heavy, and then slowly lower your sit bones toward the blankets. Your pubic bone and tailbone should be equidistant from the floor.
5. As for your hands, you can:
   a. Stack your hands in your lap, palms up.
   b. Lay them on your knees, palms down.
   c. Perform the *Anjali Mudra*: palms clasped and thumbs resting against the sternum.
6. Lengthen your tailbone down toward the ground and firm your shoulder blades into your back, making sure you don't compress your lower back.
7. Hold the pose for as long as you want, but at least for 3 minutes. If you do it regularly, alternate how you cross your legs. For example, on even-numbered days you cross your left shin in front of the right, and on odd-numbered days you do the opposite. Alternatively, you can just split practice time with one leg crossed to the other, and then the opposite.

Hero Pose

Focus: Ankles; arches; knees; thighs
Level: Beginner
Sanskrit Name: *Virasana*
Time: At least 1 minute, up to 5
Indications: Stretching; strengthening; improves digestion
Contraindications: Heart problems; headache; knee injuries; ankle injuries

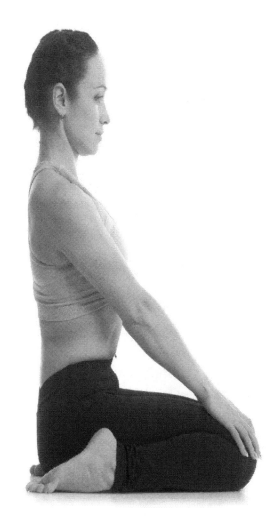

The Hero Pose is a seated pose. It stretches the thighs, knees, and ankles.

This pose is perfect for relieving tension from your legs and arches. It can even help you feel a bit better if you're having digestion issues!

To perform this exercise, you must:

1. Kneel on the ground. I recommend using a folded blanket or rug if your floor is too hard on the legs. Touch your inner knees together while keeping your thighs perpendicular to the ground.
2. Slide your feet apart, slightly wider than your hips. The tops of your feet should be flat on the floor. Try to angle your big toes slightly toward each other and press the tops of your feet evenly against the floor.
3. While you sit, your torso should lean slightly forward. Try wedging your thumbs into the backs of your knees, drawing the skin and flesh of the calf muscles gently toward your heels. Then sit down between your feet.
4. Ideally, you should rest your buttocks on the floor. If you're not comfortable doing that, a block or a thick book between your feet might do the trick.
5. Turn your thighs inward and then gently press the heads of the thigh bones into the ground with your palms.
6. Lay your hands, palms up, in your lap, one on the other. Alternatively, lay your hands on your thighs, palms down.
7. Firm your shoulder blades against your back ribs. Lift the top of your sternum. Widen your collarbones and then release your shoulder blades. Lengthen your tailbone into the floor to anchor your back.
8. To end this pose, lift your buttocks up, just above your heels, and then cross your ankles underneath. Sit back over your feet and onto the floor. Stretch your legs out in front of you.

If you're looking to add some variation to the pose, try clasping your hands together and then extending your arms forward (parallel to the ground), then turn up your palms to face the ceiling. Stretch your arms and hands thoroughly during this.

I suggest staying in this pose for at least a minute. Eventually you should stay up to five. Don't forget to control your breathing. The exercise should last as long as 3 to 9 even breaths.

Corpse Pose

Focus: Whole body
Level: Beginner
Sanskrit Name: *Savasana*
Time: At least 5 minutes
Indications: Meditation; mental relaxation; body relaxation; lowers blood pressure
Contraindications: Back injuries; back pain; late-term pregnancy

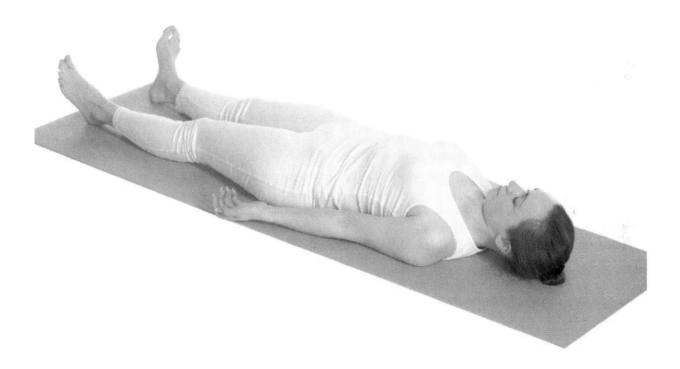

The Corpse Pose is the prime relaxation pose for beginners. I suggest you practice it a lot, even on its own, outside your typical yoga sessions.

This pose allows you to meditate, giving you the mind reconnection we all need. It relaxes the body; relieves stress; reduces both physical and mental fatigue, and even helps to lower your blood pressure.

To perform this exercise, you must:

1. Sit on the floor and bend your knees, placing your feet on the floor.
2. Lean back onto your forearms and lift your pelvis slightly off the floor.
3. Push the back of your pelvis toward the tailbone, and then lower your pelvis to the floor.
4. Extend your right leg, and then the left, pushing through your heels.
5. Release both legs, softening the groins as you do, and make sure that your legs are angled relative to the midline of your torso.
6. Narrow your front pelvis, and soften your lower back as you turn your feet out.
7. Lift the base of your skull away from the base of your neck and release the back of your neck down toward your tailbone. If you're having difficulty doing this, rest the back of your head and neck on a folded blanket.
8. Broaden the base of your skull, and then lift the crease of your neck diagonally and push it into the center of your head. Be sure your ears are equidistant from your shoulders.
9. Extend your arms up, toward the ceiling, and keep them perpendicular to the floor.
10. Sway slightly from side to side, broadening your back ribs and shoulder blades away from your spine. Release your arms, keeping them angled to the midline of your torso. Turn your arms outward, and then extend.
11. Rest the backs of your hands on the floor, keeping them as close as you can to the index finger knuckles. Spread your collarbones.
12. Now comes the hardest part: Relax! You must calm and soothe your sense organs. Clear your mind and focus on relaxing.
13. Hold the pose for 5 minutes. Performing the pose after 30 minutes of physical practice can help you get back in tune with your senses as well as functioning as a muscle relaxer.

This pose is great to open or close beginner yoga practices—but don't forget about it as you become more skilled!

Standing Half Forward Bend

Focus: Torso; back; belly
Level: Beginner
Sanskrit Name: *Ardha Uttanasana*
Time: At least 30 seconds
Indications: Stretching; strengthening; abdominal stimulation; improves pose
Contraindications: Neck injuries

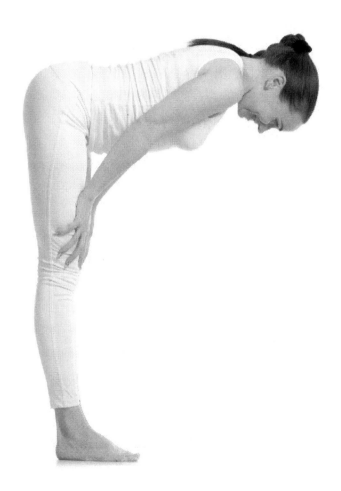

The Standing Half Forward Bend Pose is a beginner forward bend pose that stretches the front torso, strengthens the back, improves the pose, and stimulates the belly.

To perform this exercise, you must:

1. Part from the Standing Forward Bend Pose and press your palms (or fingers) into the ground beside your feet. If you can't rest your hands comfortably on the floor, use a couple of blocks as support.
2. Inhale deeply, and then fully extend your elbows, arching your torso away from your thighs, making as much distance between your pubic bone and navel as possible.
3. Use your palms (or fingers) to push down and back against the floor. Lift your sternum up and forward from the ground. Feel free to bend your knees slightly for the movement.
4. Set your head in a neutral position and gaze forward, making sure you *don't* compress the back of your neck.
5. Hold the pose for 3 to 5 breaths. End by calmly releasing your grip from the floor and coming up. The Standing Forward Bend Pose is a common follow-up for this pose.

Bound Angle Pose

Focus: Inner thighs; groins, knees
Level: Beginner
Sanskrit Name: *Baddha Konasana*
Time: At least a minute, up to 5
Indications: Strengthening; stretching; abdominal stimulation; opens hips; mental relaxation
Contraindications: Groin injury; knee injury

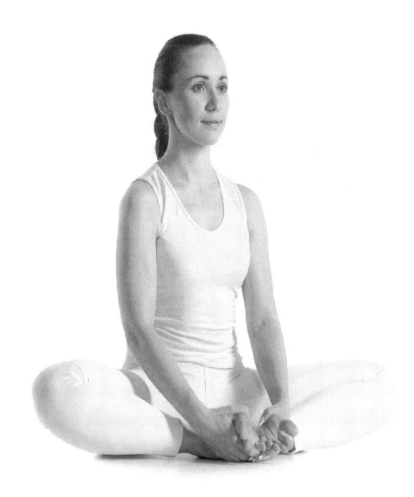

The Bound Angle Pose is a hip-opener seated pose that can stimulate the abdominal organs, heart, kidneys, and bladder.

If you've piled physical stress on your thighs, groins and knees, this pose will help you reclaim some of your wellbeing!

To perform this exercise, you must:

1. Sit on the ground with your legs stretched in front of you. Start bending your knees, pulling your heels toward your pelvis. Drop your knees out to the sides and join the soles of your feet together.
2. Bring your heels close together by pressing your soles and then bring them as close to your pelvis as you can.
3. Using your first 2 fingers and your thumb, grasp each big toe with each hand.
4. You must keep your pubis and tailbone equidistant from the floor. Firm your shoulder blades and sacrum, and then lengthen your front torso through the top of the sternum.
5. You shouldn't have to force your knees down; in fact, you must not. Pressing your thigh bones toward the floor will be enough, as your knees will follow.
6. To release this pose, lift your knees away from the floor, and then stretch your legs back to their original position.

Don't get frustrated if you're not quite getting your knees to stay grounded. It will require constant practice, but it will come eventually.

Staying anywhere from 1 to 5 minutes will be beneficial. Remember to count even breaths as you do; 3 to 9 should be fine depending on the duration.

Child Pose

Focus: Ankles; hips; thighs
Level: Beginner
Sanskrit Name: *Balasana*
Time: 30 seconds to 2 minutes
Indications: Stretching; relieving pain; mental relaxation
Contraindications: Diarrhea; pregnancy (especially late-term); knee injuries; back injuries

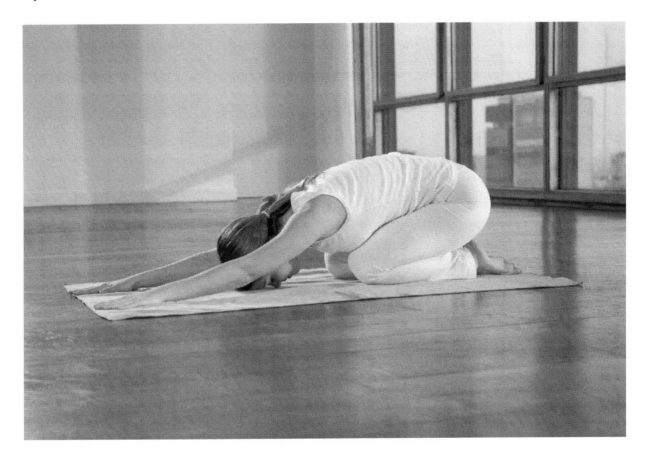

The Child Pose is a restive pose that can be performed in between other asanas in sequences.

It stretches the hips, thighs, and ankles, and it allows us to calm our mind and brain, relieving stress and fatigue. You can start this pose from the Hero Pose.

To perform this exercise, you must:

1. Kneel on the floor, touching your big toes together. Sit on your heels and then separate your knees as much as your hips will allow.
2. Exhale all the air in your lungs and then lay your torso between your thighs.
3. Broaden your sacrum across the back of your pelvis. Narrow your hip points towards your navel, nestling them down onto your inner thighs.
4. Lengthen your tailbone away from the back of your pelvis while you lift the base of your skull away from your neck.
5. Place your hands, palms up, on the floor alongside your torso. Release the fronts of your shoulders toward the floor. Let the weight of your front shoulders pull your shoulder blades across your back.
6. To end the pose, you must lengthen the front torso, and then lift from the tailbone as it presses down and into the pelvis.

The Child Pose is excellent for resting in between other asanas. Initially you might struggle to stay in it for 30 seconds, but the goal here is staying a few minutes.

Start with 30 seconds to 1 minute, but work your endurance up to 3 minutes. Count 3 to 5 even breaths, or end if you feel too strained.

If you want to increase the length of your torso during the exercise, try stretching your arms forward while lifting your buttocks slightly above and away from your heels. Extend your arms while you draw your shoulder blades down your back. Without moving your arms or hands, sit your buttocks down on your heels again.

Diamond Pose

Focus: Thighs
Level: Beginner
Sanskrit Name: *Vajrasana*
Time: At least 5 minutes, up to 15 minutes.
Indications: Meditation; improves digestion; mental relaxation
Contraindications: Joint pain

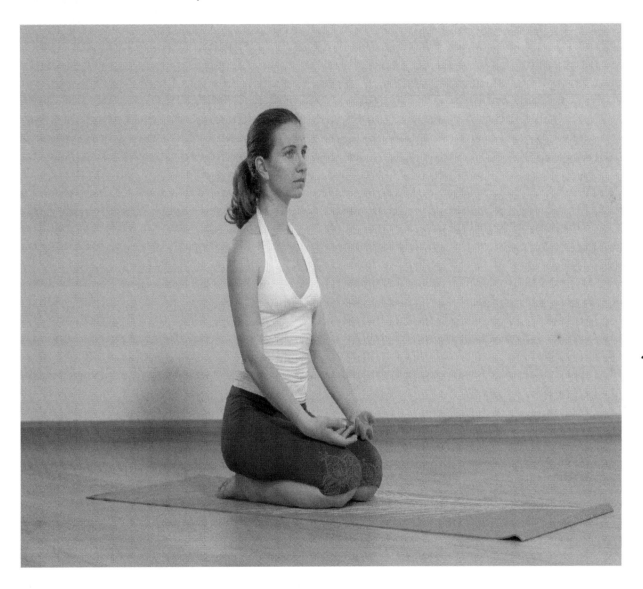

The Diamond Pose is a straightforward beginner seated pose. It is excellent for practicing breath controlling techniques (pranayama) and meditation.

It can soothe the mind; help you with gas problems; stimulate focus; and strengthen your thighs.

To perform this exercise, you must:

1. Kneel on the ground, torso upright.
2. Lower your thighs until you're sitting on the back of your shins, placing your buttocks on your feet.
3. Set your head in a neutral position, gazing forward. Make sure you keep your spine straight.
4. Close your eyes and try to concentrate *exclusively* on your breathing. Erase all thoughts that cross your mind for the moment.
5. Slowly inhale, until you can't breathe in more air, and then exhale, gently. Imagine that all your physical ailments just left your body.
6. Hold the pose for at least 3 minutes. End by opening your eyes and regaining control over your consciousness. Gradually increase your stay in this pose every time you perform it; the goal is reaching up to 15 minutes.

Practicing this pose with consistency will make your breathing better, and it will help you become more focused.

Tree Pose

Focus: Calves; ankles; spine; chest; inner thighs; shoulders
Level: Beginner
Sanskrit Name: Vrksasana
Time: 30 seconds to a minute per side
Indications: Strengthening; stretching; improves balance
Contraindications: Insomnia; high (or low) blood pressure; headache

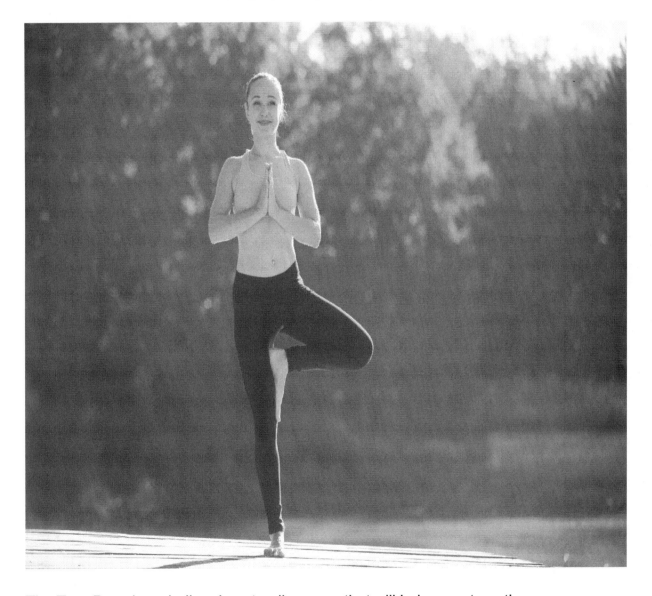

The Tree Pose is a challenging standing pose that will help you strengthen your thighs, calves, ankles, and spine.

Doing one-legged standing poses will improve your balance and reduce flat feet. It stretches the groins, inner thighs, chest, and shoulders.

To perform this exercise, you must:

1. Part from the Mountain Pose, shifting your weight subtlety onto the left foot while keeping the inner foot firmly planted on the ground.
2. Bend your right knee and reach down with your right hand to grasp your right ankle.
3. Draw your right foot up and press the sole against your inner left thigh. Try pressing your right heel into your inner left groin with your toes pointing toward the floor.
4. Lengthen your tailbone toward the floor and then raise your arms to your chest while joining your palms together in a prayer position, also known as "*Anjali Mudra*". Your thumbs should rest against your sternum.
5. Gaze at a fixed point 4 to 5 feet away with utmost concentration. Focus on your balance and stretching.
6. When ready, step back into the Mountain Pose and switch to the other leg.

Spend between 30 seconds to a minute for each side. That is the space of 1 or 2 even breaths. Alternatively, you could close your eyes instead of focusing on an object.

Garland Pose

Focus: Ankles; back; groins
Level: Beginner
Sanskrit Name: *Malasana*
Time: At least 3 minutes
Indications: Stretching; toning
Contraindications: Back injuries; knee injuries

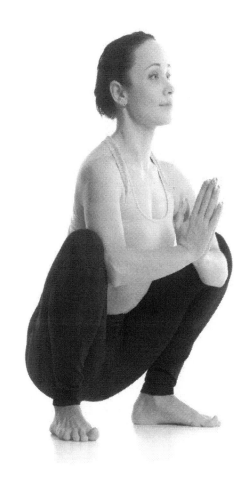

The Garland Pose is a beginner squat pose to stretch the ankles, groins and back while toning the belly.

To perform this exercise, you must:

1. Perform a deep squat with your feet as close together as you can while keeping your heels grounded. If you can't, slide a folded mat underneath.

2. Move your thighs slightly more than shoulder-width apart. Exhale and lean your torso forward, wedging it between your thighs.
3. Push your elbows against your knees and bring your palms together in the *Anjali Mudra*: Palms clasped together with your thumbs resting on your sternum.
4. Press your inner thighs against the sides of your torso, reaching your arms forward and swinging them out to the sides while you notch your shins into your armpits.
5. Press your palms into the floor or reach around your ankles and clasp them with your hands.
6. Hold the pose for 30 seconds to a minute. To come up, straighten your knees as you inhale.

Root Bond Pose

Focus: Back; spine
Level: Beginner
Sanskrit Name: *Mula Bundha*
Time: At least 3 minutes
Indications: Breathing; meditating; stretching
Contraindications: Back injuries; spine injuries

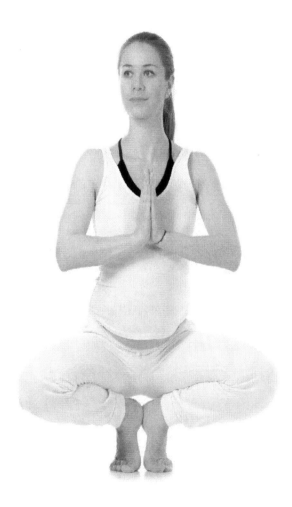

The Root Bond Pose is a powerful meditative pose that helps you train your breath retention (*pranayama*) techniques.

This pose doesn't require much physical effort, but it does require a great deal of concentration and spiritual focus. You must try to keep your body stretched without using conscious force while you try to get in tune with your own chakras.

To perform this exercise, you must:

1. Start by standing straight with your legs shoulder-width apart.
2. Raise your arms just below shoulder-level and join your palms together into a prayer position. Keep your arms firm and stretched. Close your eyes.
3. Gently crouch, placing your feet firmly against the floor.
4. Lift your heels until you're standing on your tiptoes.
5. Relax your mind and focus on your breathing.

Use the chance to train your mindfulness. Try your best to become aware of your bodily movements and sensations such as muscle tension relief, rib cage contractions, the air whistling in your ears, the temperature of your skin and so on.

It's important that you perform even-spaced breaths consciously. Ideally, you should take between 3 to 7 breaths before ending the pose, but do it as long as you can remain concentrated.

Low Lunge Pose

Focus: Thighs; groins; chest
Level: Beginner
Sanskrit Name: *Anjaneyasana*
Time: 1 to 3 minutes
Indications: Stretching; opens chest
Contraindications: Heart problems

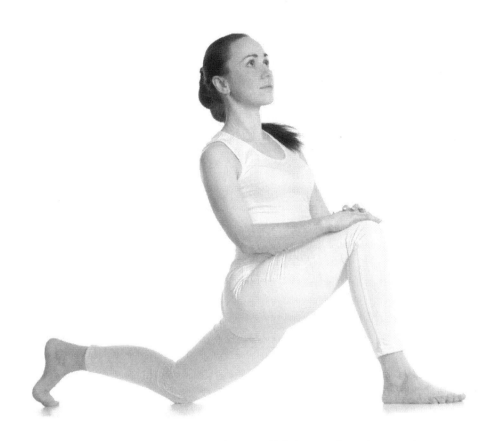

The Low Lunge Pose helps you stretch your thighs and groins and opens your chest. If you've mastered the Downward Facing Dog Pose, this pose won't be a problem!

To perform this exercise, you must:

1. Perform the Downward Facing Dog Pose.
2. Step your right foot forward between your hands, keeping your knee and your heel as aligned as possible.

3. Step your left foot back, lowering your left knee to the floor. Stretch your back until you feel comfortable. Turn the top of your left foot until your sole is perpendicular to the ground or until the top of your foot meets the floor.
4. Lift your torso until you're upright. Sweep your arms out to the sides and up until they meet. Keep them perpendicular to the floor.
5. Draw your tailbone down toward the floor and then lift your pubic bone toward your navel.
6. Bring your head back and look as far upward as you can. Be careful with your neck!
7. Once you're done holding the pose, bring back your right foot and then your left foot. Step back into the Downward Facing Dog Pose and then repeat the process on the other leg.

For starters, I recommend doing the pose *without* sweeping your arms up. If your feet aren't flexible enough, you don't have to place the tops against the floor.

Hold the pose for 3 to 5 even breaths, at least a minute. Don't forget to do each side!

Upward Facing Dog Pose

Focus: Spine; arms; wrists; shoulders; abdomen
Level: Beginner
Sanskrit Name: *Urdhva Mukha Svanasana*
Time: 15 to 40 seconds.
Indications: Stretching; strengthening; abdominal stimulation; improves pose
Contraindications: Back injuries; carpal tunnel syndrome; pregnancy (especially if late-term); headache

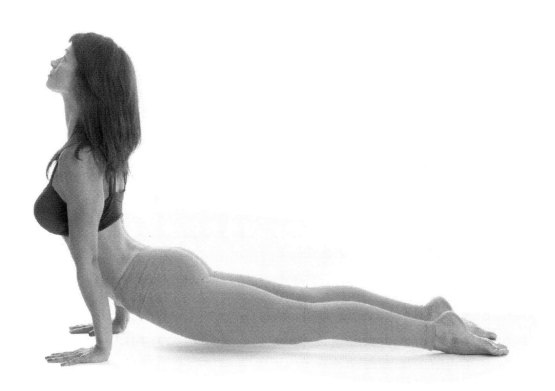

The Upward Facing Dog Pose is a challenging pose to build up endurance and open your chest.

You might've heard about it before under its more colloquial name, the *Sun Salutation Pose*. It helps both beginners and rusty yogis to warm up shoulders before action.

To perform this exercise, you must:

1. Lie flat on the ground, with your stomach facing down. Your head must be facing the floor as well.
2. Slowly bend your arms forward and rest your palms flat on the ground.
3. Gently push your arms against the floor and lift your chest off the ground.
4. Stretch your hip and thighs, leaving your feet and palms touching the floor.
5. Keep as straight as you can and look forward.
6. Optional: If you feel no discomfort during this exercise and your neck doesn't mind it, feel free to tilt your head up as much as you can.

Ideally, you should draw your shoulder blades towards one another (and down the back) and your knees should be *off* the ground.

Tilting your head back should *only* be done if you feel okay with it. There's no need to risk a potential injury!

Hold the pose for 2 to 4 even breaths. End if you feel strained or uncomfortable.

Downward Facing Dog Pose

Focus: Arms; legs; shoulders, hips; core
Level: Beginner
Sanskrit Name: *Adho Mukha Svanasana*
Time: 1 to 3 minutes.
Indications: Stretching; strengthening; building muscle
Contraindications: Carpal tunnel syndrome; late-term pregnancy; headache; high blood pressure

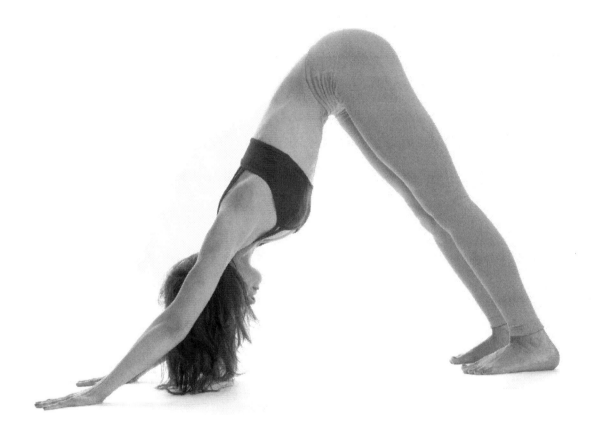

The Downward Facing Dog Pose is a celebrated core pose that stretches your shoulders, hamstrings, calves, arches, legs, arms, and hands.

It is considered as the flagship pose of yoga, and it is a well-deserved title!

It will be a bit difficult for the less flexible beginners, but that is merely an incentive to master it.

43

To perform this exercise, you must:

1. Start by standing straight with your legs shoulder-width apart.
2. Come down onto the floor on your hands and knees. You must set your knees directly below your hips, and your hands should be slightly forward of your shoulders. Rest your palms firmly against the floor.
3. Lift your knees away from the floor. Keeping your knees slightly bent will help you keep your heels planted on the floor.
4. Lengthen your tailbone away from the back of your pelvis and press lightly toward the pubis.
5. Push your top thighs back and stretch your heels toward the floor. Try to straighten your knees as much as you can, but don't lock them.
6. Firm your arms and press the bases of your index fingers into the floor.
7. Firm your shoulder blades against your back and then widen them.
8. Keep your head between your upper arms.

A partner can help you keep your heels firmly on the ground. Other than that, constantly practicing the stretching bits will help you get there on your own!

This pose serves as the basis of many different poses from beginner to advanced. It should be one of the first you master.

Hold the pose for 3 to 7 controlled breaths—usually between 1 to 3 minutes. End sooner if you feel too strained.

Three-Legged Downward Dog Pose

Focus: Arms; legs; shoulders, hips; core
Level: Beginner
Sanskrit Name: *Eka Pada Adho Mukha Svanasana*
Time: 1 to 3 minutes
Indications: Stretching; strengthening; building muscle; improving balance
Contraindications: Carpal tunnel syndrome; late-term pregnancy; headache; high blood pressure

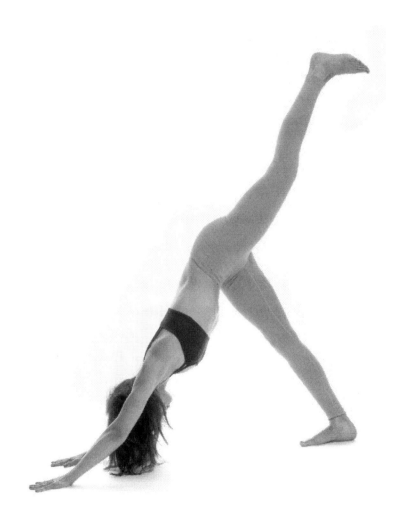

The Three-Legged Downward Dog is excellent to build up strength and muscle, especially for arms and shoulders. It allows you to stretch your legs, hips and lower body.

A fun piece of trivia: The Three-Legged Downward Dog Pose is just the Downward Facing Dog with a twist attributed to American yoga practitioners. Many poses are just modern variations from the original ones.

Constant practice of this pose will be thoroughly beneficial for your subsequent yoga sessions.

To perform this exercise, you must:

1. Start by standing straight with your legs shoulder-width apart.
2. Extend your arms to the front and then bend forward at the waist until your palms rest flat on the floor.
3. Stretch forward so that your head hangs loose between your arms.
4. Lift your right leg until it's level with your right hip. Ideally it should form a 90° angle with your left leg.
5. Optional: If you're flexible and strong enough, you might choose to lift your leg a bit more, forming a 110° or 120° angle with your left leg.

Remain relaxed and focused. Concentrate on your breathing. Hold the pose on one side for 3 to 7 breaths and then switch to the other leg and repeat.

If you feel strained at some point, feel free to switch to the other leg. The consistency and quality of your breathing will influence your comfort.

Yoga Poses for the Neck

Locust Pose

Focus: Spine; buttocks; arms; legs; belly; neck
Level: Beginner
Sanskrit Name: *Salabhasana*
Time: 30 seconds to a minute, repeated 2 to 3 times
Indications: Strengthening; stretching; improves pose; abdominal stimulation
Contraindications: Headache; back injuries; neck injuries

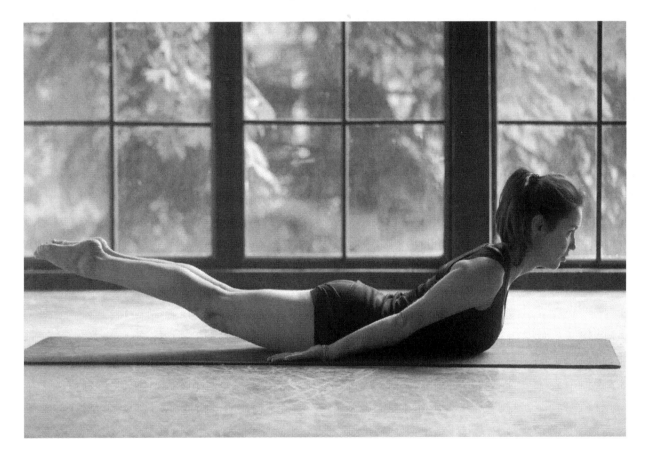

The Locust Pose is a warm-up backbend pose that helps beginners prepare for deeper stretches.

It strengthens back, legs, and arms. It might look simple, but there's more to it than meets the eye. Mastering this pose will ensure good performance in the coming backbends.

To perform this exercise, you must:

1. Optional: If your surface is too hard, I suggest you roll out a folded blanket or a rug. Otherwise you might injure your pelvis and ribs.
2. Lie on your belly with your arms resting alongside your torso. Keep your palms up and your forehead resting on the floor.
3. Turn your big toes toward each other so as to rotate your thighs. Firm your buttocks so that your coccyx presses toward your pubis.
4. Exhale the air from your lungs and then lift your upper torso, head, arms, and legs. In this exercise you will be resting on your lower ribs, belly, and pelvis.
5. Firm your buttocks, stretching your legs, first through your heels to lengthen your back legs, and then through the bases of your toes. Keep your big toes turned to each other!
6. You must keep your arms raised and parallel to the ground. Stretch back actively up to your fingertips. Imagine you have to keep a weight on your upper arms. Press your arms firmly against your back.
7. Keep your head looking forward or upward if your neck allows it.
8. End the pose if you feel too strained. Try to endure between 30 seconds and a minute.

Ideally, you should repeat this pose once or twice after ending.

Beginners might have some problems at first, but there's no need to rush. You might want to try leaving your hands, palms down, pressing into the floor to give you balance.

Holding the pose for 3 even breaths should be enough. If you're feeling too uncomfortable, end.

Warrior Pose I

Focus: Chest; shoulders; neck; belly; psoas; arms; thighs; calves; ankles; abdomen
Level: Beginner
Sanskrit Name: *Virabhadrasana I*
Time: 30 seconds to a minute per side
Indications: Strengthening; stretching
Contraindications: Heart problems; neck injuries; shoulder injuries; high blood pressure

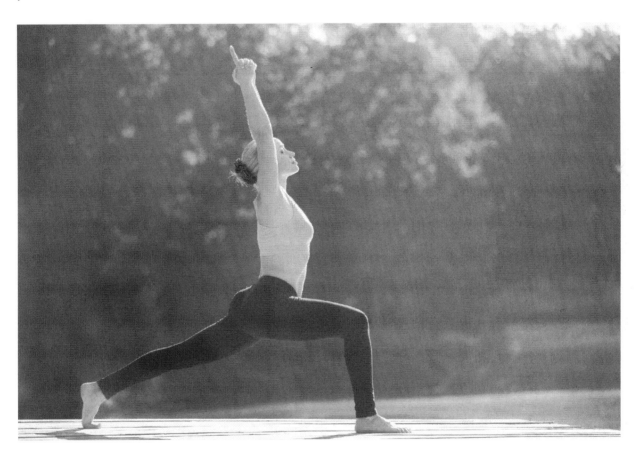

The Warrior Pose I is one of the three celebrated warrior poses of yoga.

It might strike you as silly that these yoga poses are called "warrior" poses, what with yogis being known as pacifists and all that. In this case, the name stems from the spiritual interpretation of a warrior fighting against the *universal* enemy: Self-ignorance.

In effect, the warrior poses celebrate the fight of yoga practitioners against the ultimate source of suffering.

This pose stretches the chest, lungs, shoulders, neck, belly, and groins. Constant practice will strengthen your shoulders, arms, back muscles, and calves.

To perform this exercise, you must:

1. Part from the Mountain Pose. Exhale all the air from your lungs and proceed to step your feet about 3-and-a-half or 4 feet apart.
2. Raise your arms perpendicular to the floor in opposite, parallel directions.
3. Turn your left foot 45° to 60° to the right, and your right foot 90° to the right. Align your heels, and then rotate your torso to the right. Try to square your front pelvis as much as you can.
4. If you can't keep your heels firmly planted, try pressing the head of the left femur back to the ground.
5. Lengthen your coccyx toward the floor and slightly arch your upper torso back.
6. Try to bend your right knee over your right ankle to keep the shin perpendicular to the floor. Do it as much as you can, but if you're not flexible enough you don't have to stress your body too much.
7. Lift your arms up, stretching strongly to lift your ribcage away from your pelvis. The lift should run up from your back legs, going across your whole body until it reaches your arms. Once your arms are up, bring your palms together.
8. After 30 seconds to a minute, inhale and press your heels firmly into the ground. Straighten your arms and bring them down. Take some breaths, and then switch the positioning of your legs and repeat the exercise.
9. Once you're done, step back into the Mountain Pose.

Cow Pose

Focus: Spine; torso; neck
Level: Beginner
Sanskrit Name: *Bitilasana*
Time: Up to 2 minutes, spread over all the repetitions
Indications: Stretching; abdominal stimulation
Contraindications: Neck injuries

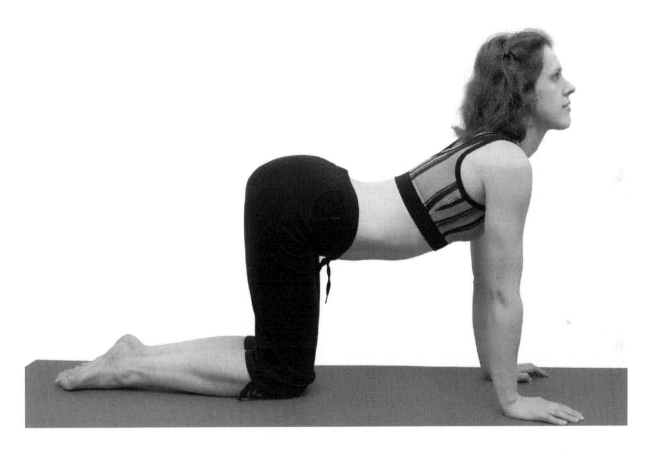

The Cow Pose is a simple pose to prepare the spine for a good yoga session. It stretches the torso, neck, and spine, as well as providing stimulation to the belly organs.

To perform this exercise, you must:

1. Get down to the floor on all fours, making sure that your knees are directly below your hips. Your wrists, elbows, and shoulders should be in line and perpendicular to the floor.
2. Position your head neutrally, staring at the floor.

3. Inhale and lift your sitting bones and chest toward the ceiling, allowing your belly to go toward the ground. Tilt your head up and look forward.
4. Exhale, and then return to the neutral "tabletop" position on all fours. Repeat between 10 and 20 times, breathing easily as you do.

If your neck is sensitive, keeping it in-line with your torso will help you, and so will broadening your shoulder blades down and away from your ears.

Cat Pose

Focus: Spine; back; neck
Level: Beginner
Sanskrit Name: *Marjaryasana*
Time: Up to 20 seconds
Indications: Stretching; abdominal stimulation
Contraindications: Neck injuries

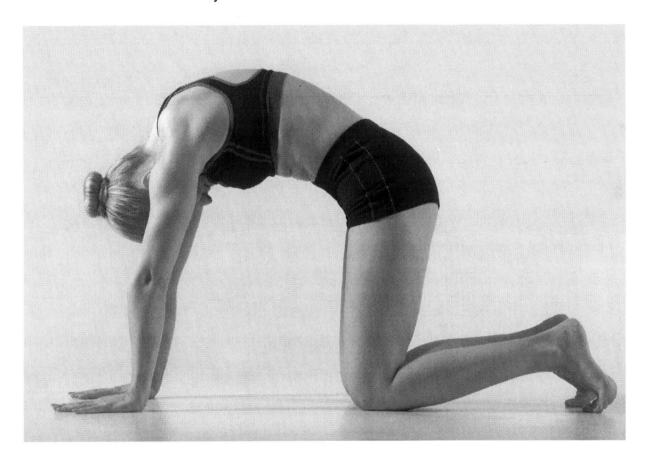

The Cat Pose is a straightforward pose to massage the spine; stretch the torso and neck, and stimulate abdominal organs.

Coupled with the Cow Pose previously covered, the Cat Pose can work miracles on your spine.

To perform this exercise, you must:

1. Go to the floor on your hands and knees, making sure that your knees are set below your hips and wrists, and that your elbows and shoulders are perpendicular to the floor.
2. Set your head in a neutral position, eyes looking down.
3. Exhale and round your spine up, just like cats do when they're rubbing against their owner's leg. Your shoulders and knees must remain in position.
4. Release your head down, but don't force your chin into your chest.
5. Inhale, and then return to the neutral "tabletop" position on your hands and knees.

I suggest you pair this pose with the Cow Pose for a deeper yoga exercise. Try performing the Cow Pose after the inhale, then the neutral position, then the Cat Pose, and so on.

A partner might come in handy if you feel like you can't round the topmost part of your back. Ask him to lay a hand between your shoulder blades to help you round it.

If your neck is strained or otherwise injured, keep it in line with the torso and try broadening your shoulder blades.

Fish Pose

Focus: Belly; neck; back; psoas
Level: Beginner
Sanskrit Name: *Matsyasana*
Time: 15 to 30 seconds
Indications: Stretching; strengthening; abdominal stimulation; improves pose
Contraindications: Back injuries; neck injuries; low (or high) blood pressure; insomnia; migraine

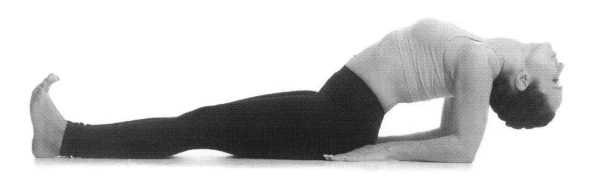

The Fish Pose is a traditional yoga pose to open the chest; stretch the psoas, intercostals, belly, neck, and back; and stimulate the belly organs.

The ancient texts define this pose as a "disease destroyer", and it has been linked with many therapeutic applications that range from menstrual pain to respiratory problems.

To perform this exercise, you must:

1. Lie prone on the floor with your knees bent, soles firmly on the ground.
2. Lift your pelvis off the floor as you inhale, just so that you can slide your hands, palms down, below your buttocks.
3. Rest your buttocks on the backs of your hands. Tuck your forearms and elbows close to the sides of your torso.
4. Press your forearms and elbows evenly into the floor, and then press your shoulder blades against your back.
5. Inhale as you lift your torso once again, bringing your head up. Then release your head down, resting the back or the crown of your head on the floor. Put next to no weight on your head to avoid neck damage.
6. Either keep your knees bent or your legs straightened. Keep your thighs pressed out through the heels if you do the latter.
7. Stay 15 to 30 seconds, breathing easily. To end, exhale and lower your torso to the floor, then draw your thighs up into your belly.

This backbend pose will serve as the basis for some advanced sequences. Avoid putting yourself in discomfort for too long, and don't be afraid to end if you feel it hurts. It takes time to master poses like these.

Bridge Pose

Focus: Chest; neck; spine; legs
Level: Beginner
Sanskrit Name: *Setu Bandha Sarvangasana*
Time: 30 seconds to a minute
Indications: Stretching; abdominal stimulation; body relaxation; improves digestion
Contraindications: Neck injuries

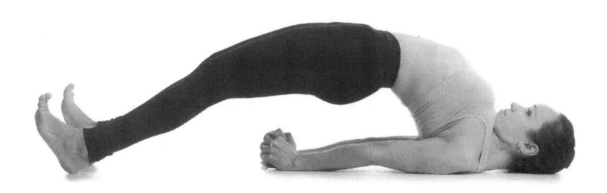

The Bridge Pose is an excellent restorative seated pose to rejuvenate the legs; stretch the chest, neck, spine; stimulate the abdominal organs and lungs; and relieve stress and fatigue.

This pose is recommended for osteoporosis, sinusitis, asthma, and high blood pressure. I suggest you roll out a thick folded blanket to soften the surface.

To perform this exercise, you must:

1. Lie prone on the floor over the blanket with your knees bent and your soles firmly planted on the ground.
2. Press your feet and arms firmly into the floor. Firm your buttocks as you lift them off the floor.
3. Keep your thighs and feet parallel.
4. Clasp your hands below your pelvis and then extend through your arms to stay on the top of your shoulders.
5. Your thighs should be parallel to the floor, and your knees should be directly over your heels.
6. Lift your pubis toward your navel while you raise your chin away from your sternum.
7. Hold the pose between 30 seconds to 1 minute. End by exhaling as you roll your spine down.

Given the weight placed on the neck and shoulders, those with neck injuries should avoid this pose.

Slide a block or bolster under your sacrum to rest your pelvis on if you're having a hard time keeping it away from the floor.

Half Lord of the Fishes Pose

Focus: Spine; shoulders; hips; neck
Level: Beginner
Sanskrit Name: *Ardha Matsyendrasana*
Time: 30 seconds to a minute per side
Indications: Stretching; stimulation; body relaxation
Contraindications: Back injuries; spine injuries

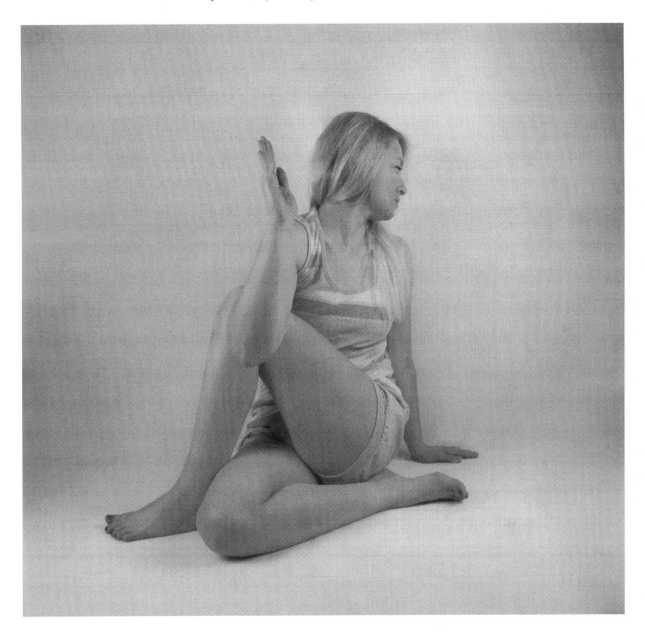

The Half Lord of the Fishes Pose is an energizing pose that stimulates the liver, kidneys, and spine; stretches the shoulders, hips and neck; and relieves fatigue and general discomfort.

I recommend rolling out a folded blanket before starting the pose.

To perform this exercise, you must:

1. Sit on the floor, legs stretched out in front of you, with your buttocks supported on the folded blanket.
2. Bend your knees, planting your soles firmly on the ground, and slide your left foot under your right leg so that it goes outside of your right hip. Lay the outside of your left leg on the ground.
3. Step your right foot over your left leg, and then stand it on the floor outside your left hip so that your right knee points directly up at the ceiling.
4. Twist toward the inside of your right thigh, and then press your right hand against the floor behind your right buttock. Set your left upper arm near your knee, outside of your right thigh. Hug your front torso and inner right thigh together.
5. Push your right foot into the ground and release your right groin. Lean your upper torso back slightly against your shoulder blades as you lengthen your tailbone to the floor.
6. Turn your head by twisting your torso to the left or to the right. With every exhale, twist a little more. Distribute your twist along your spine.
7. Hold the pose for 30 seconds to 1 minute, and then release and switch to the other side and repeat.

Supported Shoulderstand Pose

Focus: Shoulders; neck; legs; buttocks
Level: Intermediate
Sanskrit Name: *Salamba Sarvangasana*
Time: 30 seconds, up to 3 minutes
Indications: Stretching; toning; improves balance
Contraindications: Diarrhea; headache; high blood pressure; pregnancy; neck injuries

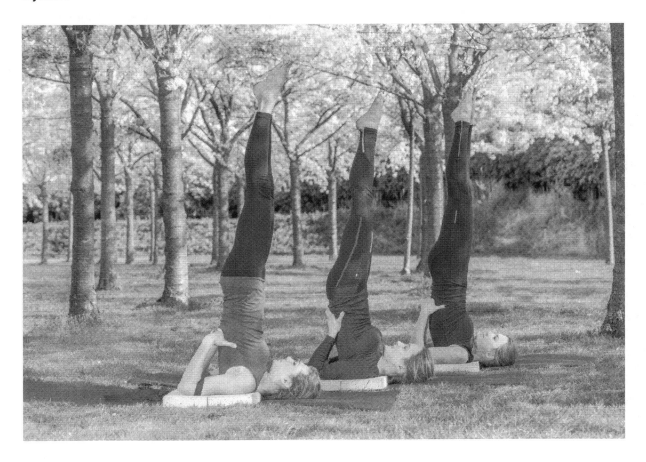

The Supported Shoulderstand Pose is an inverted yoga pose for the intermediate-advanced yogi that soothes the mind; tones the legs; stretches the shoulders and neck; and improves balance.

For this variation, fold a couple of blankets into firm rectangles and stack them on top of each other.

To perform this exercise, you must:

1. Lie on the blankets with your shoulders supported and parallel to the longer edges and your head resting on the floor.
2. Spread your arms on the floor beside your torso. Bend your knees to set your soles against the floor, heels as close as possible to your sitting bones.
3. Push your arms against the floor as you push your feet away from the ground. This will draw your thighs into your torso.
4. Initially, lift by curling your pelvis, then your back torso. Your knees should come toward your face.
5. Stretch your arms out, parallel to the edge of the blankets, and turn them out so that your fingers press into floor.
6. Bend your elbows and draw them closer. Lay the back of your upper arms on the blankets and then spread your palms against the back of your torso.
7. Lift your pelvis over your shoulders, keeping your torso somewhat perpendicular to the floor. Walk your hands up your back (toward the ground) without sliding your elbows wider than shoulder width.
8. Raise your bent knees straight up, centering your thighs with your torso and hanging your heels down by your buttocks. Push your tailbone toward the pubis and then turn your upper thighs inward slightly. Inhale and stretch your knees, pushing your heels up toward the ceiling.
9. With the backs of your legs fully lengthened, lift through your big toes so that the inner legs are a bit longer than the outer.
10. Firm your shoulder blades in your back and move your sternum toward your chin. Try keeping your forehead parallel to the floor while your chin is perpendicular. Push the backs of your upper arms and the tops of your shoulders into your blanket support to lift your spine off the ground. Gaze straight up or at your chest.
11. Start slow, holding the pose for just half a minute. Gradually increase your stay (5–10 seconds) every day or so until you become capable of enduring 3 minutes. Then continue gradually increasing until you can stay 5 minutes.
12. Come down by bending your knees into your torso, and then rolling your back carefully onto the floor with your head resting on the floor.

I advise you *not* to do this pose on your own, at least the first few times. The risks of injury are very real for those who are not yet ready for this pose.

Feathered Peacock Pose

Focus: Arms; back; shoulders; neck; chest; belly
Level: Advanced
Sanskrit Name: *Pincha Mayurasana*
Time: At least 10 seconds, up to 1 minute
Indications: Stretching; strengthening; improves balance; mental relaxation
Contraindications: Shoulder injuries; back injuries; neck injuries; headache; heart problems; high blood pressure

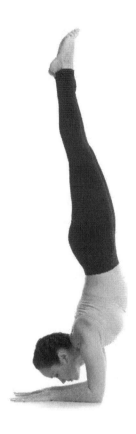

The Feathered Peacock Pose is an advanced shoulder-stand pose that strengthens the shoulders, arms, and back; stretches the shoulders, neck, chest, and belly; improves balance; and soothes the mind.

To perform this exercise, you must:

1. Part from the Downward Facing Dog Pose, near a wall, with your palms and forehead resting on the ground. Your fingertips should end right at the base of the wall.

2. Keep your forearms parallel and shoulder-width apart.
3. Firm your shoulder blades against your back torso and drag them toward your tailbone. Then rotate your upper arms outward, keeping your shoulder blades broad, and push your forearms inward. Spread your palms and push your inner wrist firmly against the floor.
4. Bend your left knee and step the foot in toward the wall. Keep your other leg active by pushing through the heel. Do a few preemptive hops before giving the final one.
5. When you do the final hop, draw your front ribs into your torso, reach your tailbone toward your heels, and slide your heels higher up the wall.
6. Drag your navel toward your spine and squeeze your outer legs together. Roll your thighs in.
7. Hold the pose for 10 to 15 seconds. Gradually work your way up to a minute. Come down one foot at a time. Be sure to switch the "kicking" leg with every practice.

Upward Lotus Pose

Focus: Arms; shoulders; neck; torso
Level: Advanced
Sanskrit Name: *Urdhva Padmasana*
Time: 30 seconds to a minute in each stage, holding the last stage up to 3 minutes
Indications: Improves balance; strengthening; stimulation
Contraindications: High blood pressure; spine injuries; elbow injuries

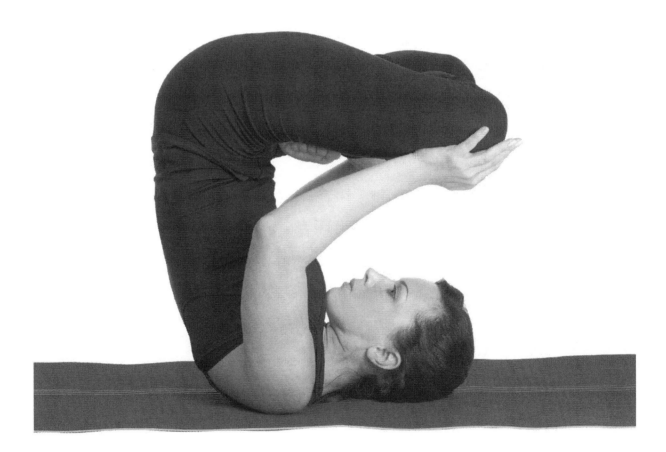

The Upward Lotus Pose is an advanced variation of the Lotus Shoulderstand pose that entails even more resistance.

It strengthens the arms, shoulders, neck, and torso muscles; improves balance and focus; and stimulates the abdominal organs.

To perform this exercise, you must:

1. Part from the Diamond Pose, and then advance into the Headstand Pose.
2. Slowly bring your legs into the lotus while consciously taking control over the balance of your body. Do this by bending your knees forward and then turning your legs outward. Bend your knees slightly toward the pelvis, and then hook your feet together.
3. Keeping your spine upright, lengthen your tailbone toward your pelvis to secure your position. Your elbows should be equidistant so that your weight is evenly distributed.
4. Balance your weight between your head, elbows, forearms, and neck.
5. Hold the pose for 30 seconds to a minute.
6. If you can, turn your pelvis and legs *slightly* to the left, and hold it for 30 seconds to a minute. You will have to shift more weight onto the right side. Now do the same but to the right side, shifting your weight to the left side.
7. Gradually increase your stay in the neutral position (not turned to either side) up to 3 minutes.

Arms, Wrists & Shoulders Yoga Poses

Upward Salute Pose

Focus: Belly; shoulders; armpits
Level: Beginner
Sanskrit Name: *Urdhva Hastasana*
Time: 30 seconds to a minute
Indications: Stretching; improves digestion; mental relaxation
Contraindications: Shoulder injuries; neck injuries

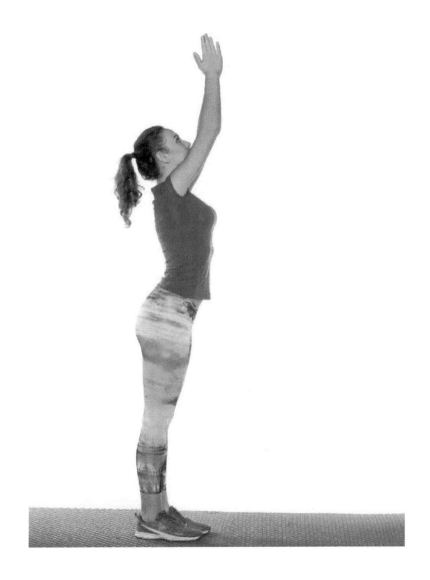

The Upward Salute Pose is a beginner standing pose that is perfect for a morning stretch or as a warm-up exercise in an expert routine.

It stretches the belly, shoulders, and armpits; improves digestion; and helps relieve the mind.

To perform this exercise, you must:

1. Part from the Mountain Pose. Turn your arms outward (or sideways) so that your palms face away from your torso, thumbs pointing backward. Inhale and sweep your arms out to the sides, and then up toward the ceiling.
2. If your shoulders are tight, stop when your arms are somewhat parallel to each other. Press your palms firmly together, if possible without hunching your shoulders forward.
3. Fully straighten your elbows, and then reach up through your pinkies, thumbs turned down toward the crown of your head. Be sure not to compress the back of your neck. Tip your head slightly and look at your thumbs.
4. Making sure that your lower front ribs *don't* protrude forward, bring your front ribs down toward your pelvis, and in toward your spine. Lengthen your tailbone toward the floor.
5. Lift your rib cage away from your pelvis, stretching the circumference of your belly.
6. Hold the pose for a few breaths. End by sweeping your arms out to the sides, and then tilting your torso forward from the hip joints. Fold into the Standing Forward Bend Pose to continue the sequence.

Cow Face Pose

Focus: Ankles; hips; thighs; shoulders; chest
Level: Beginner
Sanskrit Name: *Gomukhasana*
Time: 30 seconds to a minute per side
Indications: Stretching
Contraindications: Neck injuries; shoulder injuries

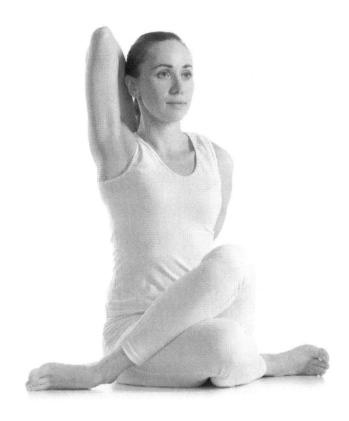

The Cow Face Pose is a challenging pose that stretches the ankles, hips, thighs, shoulders, armpits and triceps.

Perhaps you don't quite discern the cow face in the pose. Try to notice the likeliness of the crossed legs to the lips, and the bent elbows and arms to the ears.

To perform this exercise, you must:

1. Part from the Staff Pose, then bend your knees to place your feet on the ground.

2. To stack your knees, slide your left foot under the right to the outside of your right hip, then cross your right leg over the left, sliding it to the outside of your left hip.
3. Try to keep your heels equidistant to your hips while you sit evenly on your sitting bones.
4. Stretch your right arm to the right, parallel to the floor, and then rotate inward; the thumb should turn to the floor and then the wall behind you, palm facing up. Now sweep the arm behind your torso, tucking your forearm into the hollow of your lower back, in line to your waist. Your right elbow should hug the right side of your torso.
5. Roll your shoulder down to work your forearm until it's parallel to your spine. At this point your hand should be between your shoulder blades.
6. Now stretch your left arm forward, parallel to the floor. Then stretch it straight up to the ceiling, palm turned back, and lift through your left arm to bend the elbow and reach down and behind for your right hand. Hook your fingers if possible.
7. Raise your left elbow toward the ceiling while you firm your shoulder blades and lift your chest.
8. Stay in the pose for 30 seconds to a minute. Once done, release arms and uncross legs to repeat with your arms and legs reversed.

If your tight shoulders stop you from hooking your fingers, use a strap between your hands so they can pull each other.

Plank Pose

Focus: Spine; arms; wrists
Level: Beginner
Sanskrit Name: *Kumbhakasana*
Time: 30 seconds to a minute
Indications: Strengthening; toning
Contraindications: Carpal tunnel syndrome

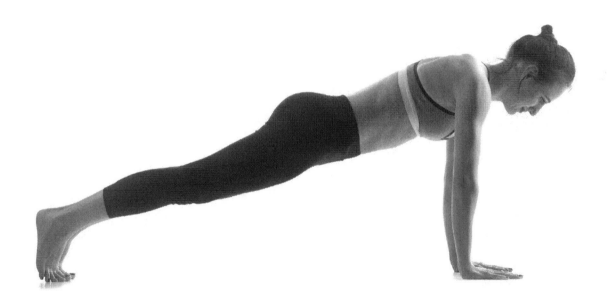

The Plank Pose is a straightforward pose that helps beginner yogis strengthen the arms, wrists, and spine in anticipation of more challenging poses.

To perform this exercise, you must:

1. Part from the Downward Facing Dog Pose. Inhale and push your torso forward until your arms are perpendicular to the floor, your shoulders are directly over your wrists, and your torso is parallel to the ground.

2. Push your outer arms inward, firming the bases of your index fingers into the floor. Adjust your shoulder blades against your back, then spread them away from your spine as you move your collarbones away from your sternum.
3. Push your front thighs toward the ceiling, resisting your tailbone toward the ground as you lengthen it toward your heels. Raise the base of your skull away from the back of your neck and stare down to the floor.
4. Hold the pose between 30 to seconds to 1 minute.

Four Limbed Staff Pose

Focus: Abdomen; arms; wrists
Level: Beginner
Sanskrit Name: *Chaturanga Dandasana*
Time: 10 to 30 seconds
Indications: Strengthening; toning
Contraindications: Carpal tunnel syndrome; late-term pregnancy

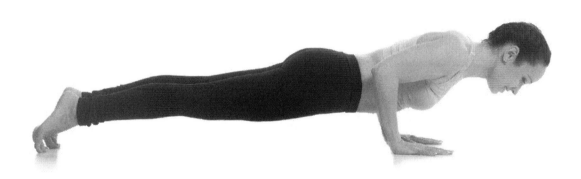

The Four Limbed Staff Pose is a step-up (or technically step-down) of the Staff Pose that helps beginners strengthen the arms, abs, and wrists.

To perform this exercise, you must:

1. Part from the Downward Facing Dog Pose, and then perform the Plank Pose.
2. Firm your shoulder blades against your back ribs, and then push your tailbone toward your pubis.

3. Lower your torso and legs to just a few inches above and parallel to the floor. If your lower back rocks toward the floor and your tailbone sticks toward the ceiling, steady your position by firmly keeping your tailbone in place and your legs active and turned to the inside. Pull your pubis toward your navel.

4. Keep your shoulder blades broad, and don't let your elbows spread out to the sides; you must hold them into the sides of your torso and then pull them toward your heels.

5. Push the bases of your fingers into the floor, and then lift the top of your sternum. Keep your head looking forward.

6. Hold this pose for 10 to 30 seconds, take a few breaths, and then come up. Alternatively, step back into the Downward Facing Dog Pose, lifting through your top thighs and tailbone.

Dolphin Plank Pose

Focus: Shoulders; hamstrings; calves; arches; legs; arms
Level: Intermediate
Sanskrit Name: *Makara Adho Mukha Svanasana*
Time: 30 seconds to a minute
Indications: Stretching; strengthening
Contraindications: Shoulder injuries; neck injuries

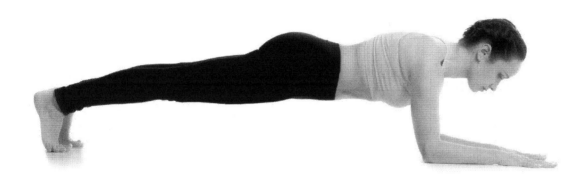

The Dolphin Plank Pose is a variation of the Dolphin Pose that strengthens and stretches the shoulders, hamstrings, calves, arms, and legs.

The focus of this pose is on strengthening, not balancing. It is great to build up endurance for the following, more challenging, poses.

To perform this exercise, you must:

1. Part from the Dolphin Pose, keeping your knees bent initially.
2. Walk your feet back, right until your shoulders are located directly above your elbows and your torso is parallel to the floor.
3. Push your elbows and inner forearms against the floor. Firm your shoulder blades against your back, and then spread them away from your spine. Spread your collarbones away from your sternum.
4. Push your front thighs toward the ceiling and lengthen your tailbone toward the heels. Move the base of your skull up and away from the back of your neck, and keep a neutral gaze toward the floor.
5. Hold the pose between 30 seconds to a minute. End by calmly releasing your knees to the floor as you exhale.

Upward Plank Pose

Focus: Arms; wrists; shoulders; legs; chest; ankles
Level: Intermediate
Sanskrit Name: *Purvottanasana*
Time: 20 to 40 seconds
Indications: Stretching; strengthening
Contraindications: Wrist injuries; neck injuries

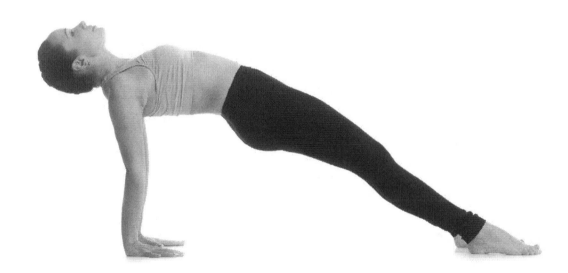

The Upward Plank Pose is yet another variation of the Plank Pose that strengthens the arms, wrist, and legs, just as it stretches the pectorals, shoulders, and ankles.

To perform this exercise, you must:

1. Part from the Staff Pose, placing your hands many inches behind your hips, with your fingertips pointing forward.
2. Bend your knees and rest your feet on the floor, big toes turned back, facing inward, with your heels a foot or so away from your buttocks.

3. Breathe easily and press your inner feet and hands into the ground, lifting your hips until you reach a reverse "tabletop" position (on all fours but with your belly facing toward the ceiling). Your torso and thighs should be somewhat parallel to the floor, just like your shins and arms are perpendicular.
4. Keep the height of your hips, and then extend and stretch your legs, one at a time.
5. Lift your hips a bit higher, but keep your buttocks soft.
6. Push your shoulder blades against the back of your torso, supporting the lift of your chest.
7. Without compressing the base/back of your neck, drop your head back.
8. Hold the pose between 20 and 40 seconds, breathing easily. End by sitting back in the Staff Pose.

Side Plank Pose

Focus: Arms; belly; legs; wrists; legs
Level: Intermediate
Sanskrit Name: *Vasisthasana*
Time: 15 to 30 seconds per side
Indications: Stretching; strengthening; improves balance
Contraindications: Wrist injuries; elbow injuries; shoulder injuries

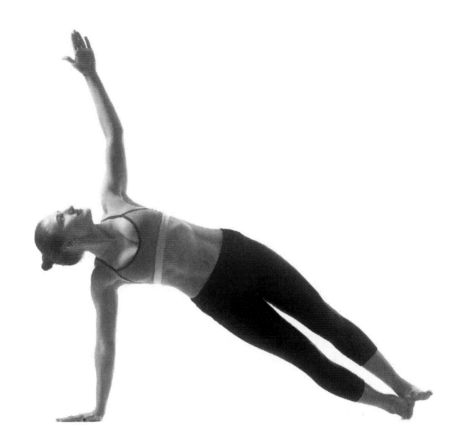

This Side Plank Pose is the meaner cousin of the Plank Pose. It takes it to the next level by turning the pose into an arm balance pose that will train your arms and wrists in preparation for the coming challenges.

To perform this exercise, you must:

1. Part from the Downward Facing Dog Pose, but then move onto the outside edge of your right foot and stack your left foot on top of the right. Now swing your left hand onto your left hip, turning your torso to the right as you do.
2. Shift the weight of your body onto the outer left foot and left hand.

3. The supporting hand *shouldn't* be directly under the shoulder; instead, position it slightly in front thereof so that the supporting arm is a bit angled relative to the floor.
4. Straighten the arm by firming the triceps muscle, and then push the base of the index finger into the floor.
5. Firm your shoulder blades and sacrum against your back torso. Harden your thighs and push through your heels down toward the ground. Align your entire body into a long diagonal line from heels to crown.
6. You can stretch your top arm toward the ceiling, parallel to the shoulder line. Keep your head in a neutral position, or gaze at the top hand.
7. Hold the pose for 15 to 30 seconds, and then step back into the Downward Facing Dog Pose. Take a few breaths, and then repeat on the other side for the same length of time.

Upward Bow Pose

Focus: Chest; arms; wrists; legs; buttocks; spine
Level: Intermediate
Sanskrit Name: *Urdhva Dhanurasana*
Time: 5 to 10 seconds, 3 to 10 times
Indications: Stretching; strengthening; stimulation; opens chest
Contraindications: Carpal tunnel syndrome; back injuries; diarrhea; headache; heart problems; low (or high) blood pressure

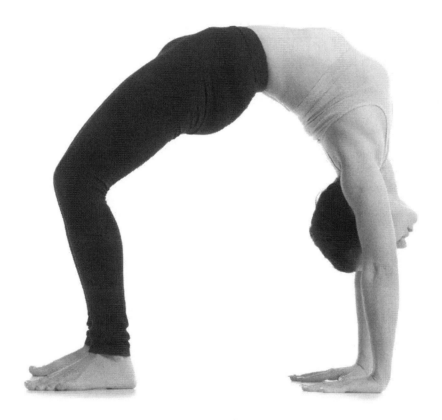

The Upward Bow Pose is a daring chest opener pose that stretches the chest and lungs; strengthens the arms, wrists, legs, buttocks, and spine; boosts stamina; and stimulates the thyroid and pituitary glands.

To perform this exercise, you must:

1. Lie prone on the ground, bending your knees to set your soles on the floor. Your heels should be near to your sitting bones.

81

2. Stretch your arms up toward the ceiling and then bend your elbows back to spread your palms on the floor beside your head. Your forearms should be somewhat perpendicular to the floor, with your fingers pointing toward your shoulders.
3. Firmly press your feet against the floor, and then push your tailbone up toward your pubis. Firm your buttocks as you lift them off the floor, keeping your thighs and inner feet parallel.
4. Take a couple of breaths. Now press your hands into the floor and drag your shoulder blades against your back to lift onto the crown of your head. Take a couple of breaths while keeping your arms parallel.
5. Press your feet and hands against the floor as you drag your tailbone and shoulder blades up against your back to lift your head off the floor. Straighten your arms and turn your thighs up to lift your pubis toward your navel.
6. The weight should be directed toward the bases of your index fingers. Broaden your shoulder blades across your back and let your head hang.
7. Hold the pose for 5 to 10 seconds, breathing evenly. End the pose and repeat 3 to 10 times.

If you're having problems performing the backbend because of your armpits and/or groins, use a support, like a pair of stacked books or a block, below your hands or feet.

Shoulder-Pressing Pose

Focus: Arms; wrists; belly
Level: Advanced
Sanskrit Name: *Bhujapidasana*
Time: 30 to 40 seconds
Indications: Strengthening; improves balance; toning
Contraindications: Wrist injuries; shoulders injuries; back injuries; elbow injuries

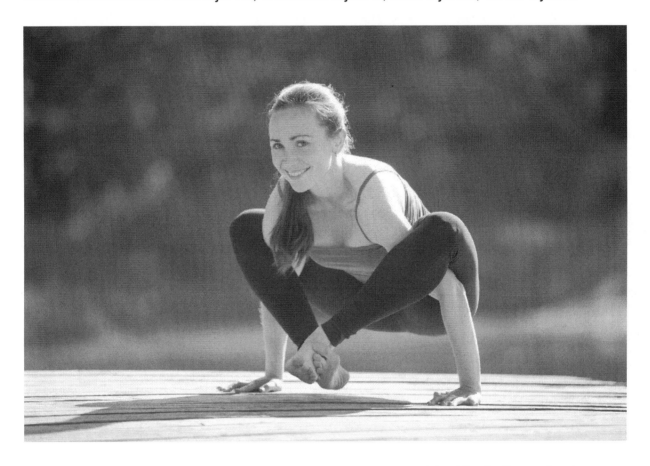

The Shoulder-Pressing Pose is a slightly simpler version of the Firefly Pose. It requires you to use precise positioning and strength. It strengthens the arms and wrist, tones the belly, and improves balance.

To perform this exercise, you must:

1. Start by squatting with your feet a bit closer than shoulder-width apart, knees wide.
2. Tilt your torso forward, wedging it between your inner thighs. Keeping your torso low, raise your hips until your thighs are nearly parallel to the floor.

3. Nestle your left upper arm and shoulder under the back of your left thigh, above the knee, and rest your left hand on the floor outside the edge of your left foot, fingers pointing forward. Do the same on the other side, rounding your upper back in the process.
4. Push your inner hands evenly into the floor, and slowly sway your weight back and off your feet, onto your hands. Straighten your arms while your feet lift slightly off the ground. This is the product of shifting your center of gravity, not just strength.
5. Snuggle your outer arms with your inner thighs, crossing your right ankle over your left ankle. Keep your head in a neutral position, looking forward.
6. Hold the pose for 30 to 40 seconds. Come up by bending your elbows and then releasing your feet back to the ground.

Crane Pose

Focus: Arms; wrists; abdomen
Level: Advanced
Sanskrit Name: *Bakasana*
Time: 20 seconds to 1 minute
Indications: Strengthening; improves balance
Contraindications: Carpal tunnel syndrome; wrist injuries; pregnancy

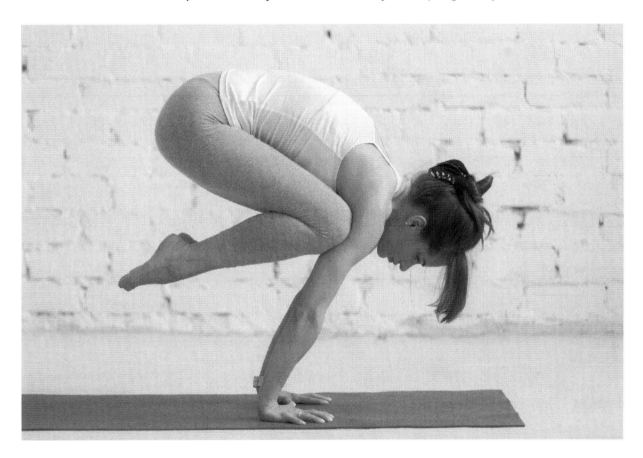

The Crane Pose is a tough pose that strengthens the arms, wrists, and abs. It demands a lot of physical strength, balance, and wrist resistance.

To perform this exercise, you must:

1. Part from the Mountain Pose. Then squat down, keeping your inner feet a few inches apart. If you can't ground your heels completely on the floor, slide a folded blanket underneath.
2. Separate your knees a little wider than your hips and bend your torso forward, wedging it between your inner thighs.

3. Stretch your arms forward and then bend your elbows, resting your hands on the ground while the backs of your upper arms rest against your shins.
4. Nestle your inner thighs to the sides of your torso, tuck your shins into your armpits, and then slide your upper arms as low onto your shins as you can. Raise up onto the balls of your feet and lean forward a little more, shifting the weight of your torso to the backs of your upper arms.
5. Keep your tailbone as close to your heels as possible to round your back as much as you can.
6. Lean forward again until your torso and legs remain balanced on the backs of your upper arms. If this is your first time doing the Crane Pose, it's best if you remain secured on top of your bent arms.
7. To progress, you must squeeze your legs against your arms, pushing your inner hands firmly to the floor as you straighten your elbows. Your arms should be angled slightly forward to the floor.
8. Your inner knees should be snuggled to your outer arms near the armpits. Keep your head in a neutral position, looking to the floor or straight forward.
9. Hold the pose between 20 seconds and a minute. End by exhaling and slowly lowering your feet to the ground, stepping back into the squat.

This pose is generally difficult to perform and even harder to master. Train with patience and don't be afraid of using blocks, bolsters, or any kind of support to help you lift off the floor.

Side Crane Pose

Focus: Arms; wrists; spine
Level: Advanced
Sanskrit Name: *Parsva Bakasana*
Time: 20 to 40 seconds per side
Indications: Strengthening; improves balance
Contraindications: Wrist injuries; back injuries

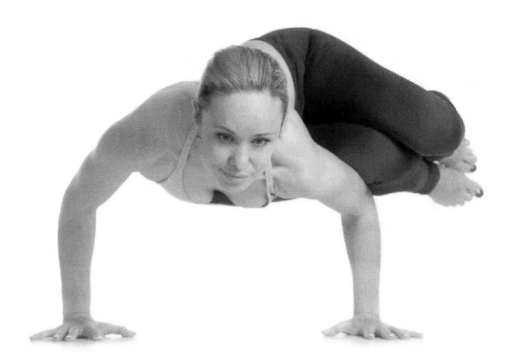

The Side Crane Pose is the advanced variation of the normal Crane Pose, requiring even more strength and balance. It strengthens the arms, wrists, and spine, and improves your sense of balance.

To perform this exercise, you must:

1. Start from a standing position, and then bend your knees into a half-squat, keeping your thighs parallel to the floor. If your heels aren't firmly grounded, slide a folded blanket or bolster underneath.

2. Bring your left elbow to the outside of your right thigh as you soften your belly. While exhaling deeply, rotate your torso to the right and bring your left lower ribs across your right thigh as far as you can.

3. Move the back of your left arm down the outside part of your right thigh, bringing the outer armpit as close to the outer thigh as possible. Keep your arm in place and do a slight back bend to drag your shoulder, increasing the twist of your torso.

4. Repeat these alternating backbend movements, exhale by exhale, until you reach maximum rotation. Then slide your left upper arm a few inches toward your right hip, pressing it firmly against your right thigh. Maintaining this pressure, drag the upper arm back toward your right knee, making sure that your skin doesn't slide, to lock it in place.

5. Squat down fully, keeping your buttocks *just* above your heels. Place your left palm on the floor beside your right foot. If your hand doesn't reach the ground, try tipping your torso to the right until you can rest the palm down. Keep the contact, and then lean to the right to place your right hand.

6. At this point, both hands should be shoulder-width apart and your weight should be shifted onto your feet.

7. Focus on keeping the contact between your left arm and right thigh while slowly lifting your pelvis, then moving it to the right. The goal is wedging the middle of your abdomen above and between your hands. Finding the *perfect* position is up to how you feel. The weight on your hands should increase just as it decreases on your feet.

8. Keep your feet together and push through the inner edges. Draw your heels toward your buttocks and soften your belly in anticipation for the twist. Firmly pull your left hip down and lift both feet up. Your arms may be slightly bent, so straighten as much as you can without letting your legs go down.

9. Fully straighten your right arm and, as you lift your right shoulder, twist your spine further. Raise your chest and head and then gaze forward. Breathe easily, holding the pose for 20 to 40 seconds. Repeat on the other side for the same length of time.

For newcomers, using a block or bolster to lower your head on to as you lift your feet off the floor will help you keep your balance.

Firefly Pose

Focus: Inner groins; back; arms; wrists; belly
Level: Advanced
Sanskrit Name: *Tittibhasana*
Time: 15 to 30 seconds
Indications: Stretching; strengthening; improves balance; toning
Contraindications: Wrist injuries; shoulders injuries; back injuries; elbow injuries

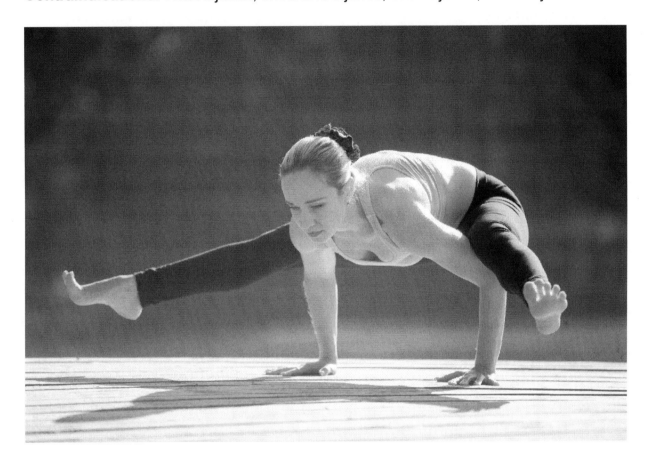

The Firefly Pose is an exciting pose that demands a great deal of strength. It stretches the inner groins, back torso, arms, and wrists; tones the belly; improves sense of balance; and builds strength.

To perform this exercise, you must:

1. Start by squatting with your feet a little less than shoulder-width apart. Tilt your pelvis forward and drag your trunk between your legs. Keep it low as you straighten your legs enough to lift your pelvis to knee height.

2. Bring your left upper arm and shoulder as far as you can below the back of your left thigh, and then place your left hand on the ground outside the side of your foot, fingers pointing forward. Do the same on the other side.
3. Lift from the floor by shifting your center of gravity. Push your hands into the floor and slowly sway your weight back off your feet and onto your hands. Keep your inner thighs as high on your arms as you can.
4. Stretch your legs out to the sides, keeping them as straight as possible. The goal is keeping your pelvis high to make your legs parallel to the floor.
5. Push through the bases of your toes while you pull your toes themselves toward your torso and spread them evenly. The edges of your inner feet should be angled forward.
6. Extend your arms as long as you can, and then hollow your chest while you spread your shoulder blades. This will help you round your upper back to lift your torso.
7. Keep your neck soft and your head looking forward. Breathe easily and hold the pose for 15 to 30 seconds.

If the pose seems a bit too hard for you but you still want to try, try placing two blocks to elevate each heel while you lift your pelvis from the floor.

Pose Dedicated to the Sage I

Focus: Arms; wrists; belly; spine
Level: Advanced
Sanskrit Name: *Eka Pada Koundinyanasana I*
Time: 20 to 40 seconds per side
Indications: Strengthening; toning
Contraindications: Wrist injuries; back injuries

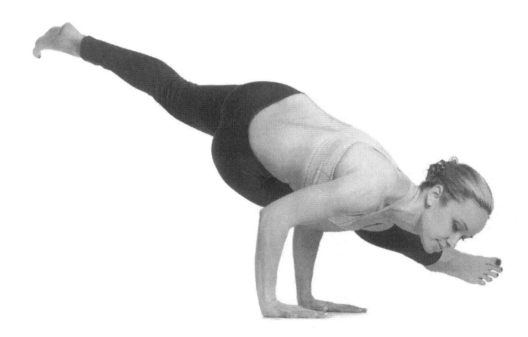

The Pose Dedicated to the Sage Koundinya I Pose is a complex pose that involves a lot of strength in the arms and wrists. It thoroughly strengthens and tones the arms, wrists, belly, and spine.

To perform this exercise, you must:

1. Part from the Mountain Pose, then bend your knees as if you were trying to squat, but take your left knee to the floor. Turn your left foot so it points to the right. Sit on the heel.

2. Cross your right foot over your left thigh and rest it firmly on the ground, sole down, beside your left knee. At this point your right knee should point toward the ceiling.

3. To perform the twist, you must bring your left side (waist, ribs, and shoulder) around to the right. Place your left upper arm across your right thigh, sliding it to your left outer armpit, down the outside of the thigh.

4. You will have to perform movements like those utilized in the Side Crane Pose to potentiate your twist. This will help you nestle your left upper arm and right outer thigh. The trick is keeping the contact high on the arm and far to the outside of the thigh.

5. Straighten your left elbow and put your left palm down on the ground. To do this you might have to lean to the right. To place your right hand, you will have to carefully lift both hips, without losing your thigh placement; do this by leaning to the right.

6. At this point, your hands should be shoulder-width apart, with your middle fingers parallel to each other. Your weight should still be shifted onto your knees and feet.

7. Lift your hips so that you can flip your left foot to stand heel-up, then lift your left knee off the floor so most of your weight is on your feet. Raise your hips a little higher to shift part of the weight to your torso, bringing it down between your hands, midline centered with your middle fingers.

8. Lean your weight a bit forward, bend your left elbow, then tilt your head and shoulders a bit toward the ground. This way you leverage your right foot up, and then you can lean your weight forward until your left foot becomes lighter. Exhale and lift it up.

9. To complete, straighten both your knees with an inhale. Lift the left leg until it's parallel to the floor, bend your left elbow, then lift your right foot higher. Adjust the height of your right shoulder so that it's in line with the left, and then bring your torso parallel to the ground.

10. Hold the pose for 20 to 40 seconds, breathing easily. Don't forget to repeat on the other side for the same time.

Pose Dedicated to the Sage II

Focus: Arms; wrists; belly; spine
Level: Advanced
Sanskrit Name: *Eka Pada Koundinyanasana II*
Time: 20 to 40 seconds per side
Indications: Strengthening; toning
Contraindications: Wrist injuries; back injuries

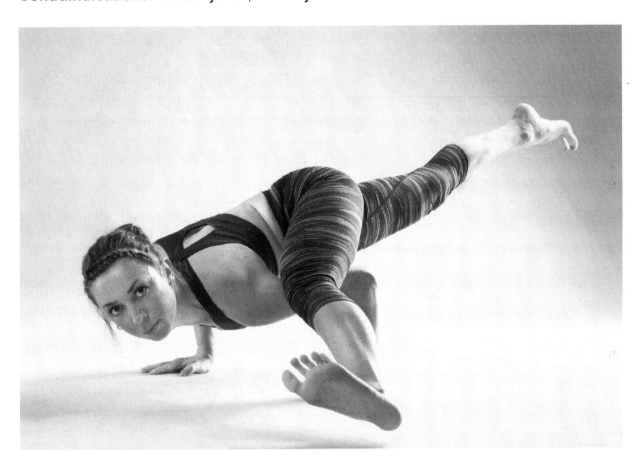

The Pose Dedicated to the Sage Koundinya II is the continuation of the previous one. It likewise involves a lot of strength in the arms and wrists, and strengthens and tones the arms, wrists, belly, and spine.

To perform this exercise, you must:

1. Part from the Downward Facing Dog Pose with your hands shoulder-width apart.

2. Step your left foot forward, past the outside of your left arm, and rest it on the floor in front of your left hand.
3. Bend your left elbow and rotate your torso to the right, dropping your left shoulder and torso as low as you can on your inner left thigh.
4. Push your thigh toward your torso and slide your left upper arm and shoulder as far as possible underneath the back of your left thigh, just above the knee. Move the back of your thigh as high as you can on your upper arm.
5. Keeping your weight centered in between your hands, start to creep your left foot forward along the ground so more weight shifts from your leg to your arm. Your left foot will naturally move a little to the left.
6. The moment you can't walk your foot farther without lifting it, straighten your knee as much as possible, reaching the foot forward and out to the left side.
7. Bend both elbows and shift your weight far between your hands until you can lift your back leg.
8. Lift strongly to make the leg parallel to the floor. With the knee extended, push straight back through your foot.
9. Raise your chest until your torso is parallel to the floor and push down through your inner hands to help keep this position.
10. Lift your head and gaze forward.
11. Breathing easily, hold the pose for 20 to 40 seconds. Step back into the Downward Facing Dog Pose, and then repeat on the other side.

Eight Angle Pose

Focus: Torso; wrists; arms; abdomen
Level: Advanced
Sanskrit Name: *Astavakrasana*
Time: 30 seconds to a minute per side
Indications: Strengthening; toning
Contraindications: Wrist injuries; elbow injuries; shoulder injuries

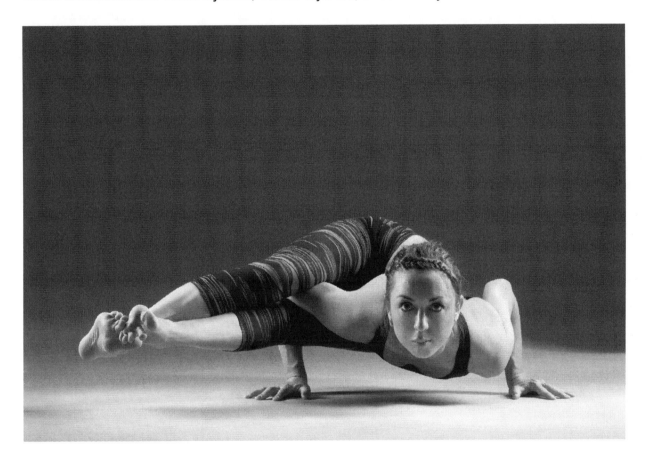

The Eight Angle Pose is an advanced arm balance pose that strengthens the torso, wrists, and arms, and tones the abdominal muscles.

1. Part from the Mountain Pose, and separate your feet a little less than shoulder-width.
2. Bend into the Standing Forward Bend Pose, push your hands into the floor outside your feet, and then slip your right arm to the inside and behind your right leg. Continue pressing the hand onto the floor outside your right foot.
3. Move your right arm across the back of your right knee, until your knee is up on the back of your right shoulder.

4. Prop your shoulder against your knee and slide your left foot to the right. Cross your left ankle in front of the right, and then hook your ankles. Lean a bit to left, shifting part of the weight off your left arm, and begin to lift your feet a few inches off the floor.

5. While supporting your right leg on the shoulder, bend your elbows. Tilt your torso forward to make it parallel to the floor and, as you tilt it, straighten your knees and stretch your legs out to the right, making them parallel to the floor and perpendicular to your torso.

6. Wedge your upper right arm between your thighs, and with the pressure, twist your torso to the left. Keeping your elbows close to your torso, gaze down toward the floor.

7. Hold the pose for 30 seconds to a minute. Come down by slowly straightening your arms down and lifting your torso back to upright. Bend your knees, unhook your ankles, and return your feet to the floor. Step back into the Standing Forward Bend Pose, take a few breaths, and repeat on the other side.

Peacock Pose

Focus: Wrists; forearms; back; legs; abdomen
Level: Advanced
Sanskrit Name: *Mayurasana*
Time: 10 to 30 seconds
Indications: Strengthening; toning
Contraindications: Wrist injuries; elbow injuries

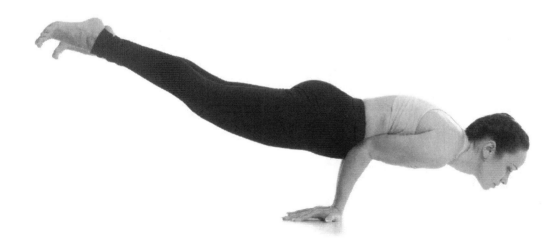

The Peacock Pose is a tough arm balance pose that symbolizes the peacock.

This pose is great for strengthening the wrists, forearms, back muscles, and legs, and for toning the abdomen.

To perform this exercise, you must:

1. Kneel on the floor, keeping your knees wide, and sit on your heels.
2. Lean forward and push your palms into the floor with your fingers turned back toward your torso (thumbs pointing to the sides).

3. Slightly bend your elbows and prop the pinky sides of your hands and the outer forearms together. Bend your elbows again to form a right angle, and then slide your knees to the outside of your arms and forward of your hands.
4. Rest your front torso on the backs of your upper arms, and then brace your belly onto your elbows.
5. Optional: If your elbows are sliding apart, you can use a strap to bind them together. Simply position the strap *just* above your elbows.
6. Firm your belly against the pressure of your elbows and lower your forehead into the ground. Now straighten your knees and stretch your legs out behind your torso, resting the tops of your feet on the floor. Slightly harden your buttocks and round your shoulders down.
7. Lift your head off the ground and gaze forward. Shift your weight slowly forward to lever your feet off the floor. Your torso and legs should be somewhat parallel to the floor.
8. At first, hold the pose for 10 seconds or so. Gradually increase your stay as you gain experience, up to 30 seconds.

Handstand Pose

Focus: Shoulders; arms; wrists; belly
Level: Advanced
Sanskrit Name: *Adho Mukha Vrksasana*
Time: 10 seconds to a minute
Indications: Stretching; strengthening; improves balance
Contraindications: Back injuries; shoulder injuries; headache; heat problems; high blood pressure; pregnancy

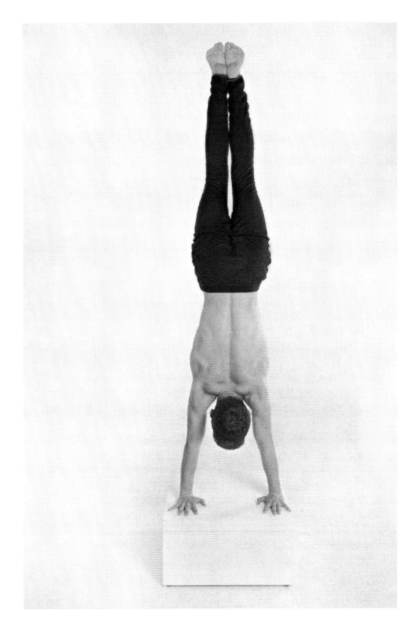

The Handstand Pose is an inverted pose that demands focus, strength and sense of balance. It strengthens the shoulders, arms, and wrists; stretches and tones the belly; improves sense of balance; and helps calm the brain.

To perform this exercise, initially propped against a wall, you must:

1. Part from the Downward Facing Dog Pose, keeping your fingertips an inch or more away from the wall. Keep your hands shoulder-width.
2. If your shoulders are tight, try turning your index fingers out; if not, arrange them parallel to each other. If you feel a little scared about performing this pose, don't worry! It's the instinct of wanting to avoid falling.
3. Secure yourself for the headstand by firming your shoulder blades against your back torso, and then lengthen them toward your tailbone.
4. Rotate your upper arms outward, keeping your shoulder blades broadened, and nestle your outer arms inward.
5. Spread your palms and push the bases of your index fingers firmly against the ground.
6. Bend your left knee and step your left foot in toward the wall. Keep the other (the right) leg active by pushing through the heel. Take a few short hops before you take the final leap upside down.
7. Sweep your right leg through a wide arc to the wall as you kick your left foot off the floor, pushing through the heel to straighten the left knee. With both legs off the ground, use your deep core abdominal muscles to help you lift your hips over your shoulders.
8. Keep doing these hops until you build sufficient strength to kick yourself all the way into the pose. Initially you might slam your heels against the wall, but as you become more skilled you'll be able to do it more elegantly.
9. If you feel that your armpits and groins become tight, it might stem from your lower back being too compressed. Lengthen this area by drawing your front ribs into your torso, and then reaching your tailbone toward your heels. Try sliding your heels higher up the wall and snuggling your outer legs together, rolling your thighs in as you do.
10. Hang your head between your shoulders blades and gaze back to the center of the room.
11. Initially, try holding this pose for 10 to 15 seconds, breathing easily and fully. Gradually increase your stay in 5-second increments until you reach a whole minute.
12. To come down, try to keep your shoulder blades up and broad, and bring one foot down at a time. You might want to try switching your "kick" leg every time you practice this pose.

Side Hand to Toe Plank Pose

Focus: Arms; belly; legs; wrists; legs; core
Level: Advanced
Sanskrit Name: *Vasisthasana*
Time: 30 seconds to a minute per side, up to 2 minutes
Indications: Stretching; strengthening; improves balance; toning
Contraindications: Wrist injuries; elbow injuries; shoulder injuries; ankle injuries

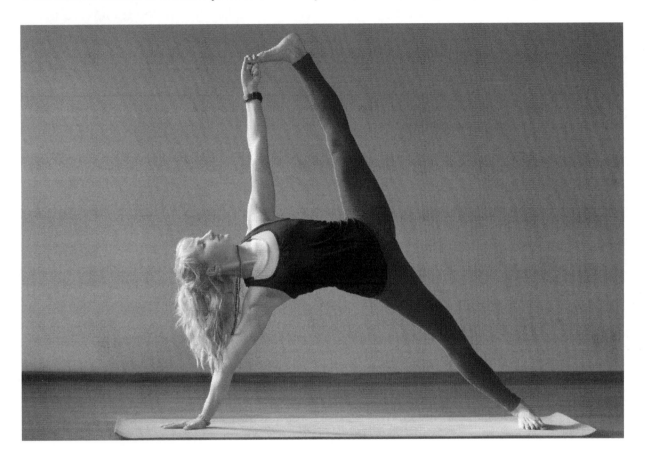

The Side Hand to Toe Plank Pose is an advanced variation of the already-challenging Side Plank Pose.

Besides the benefits of the Side Plank Pose, this variation improves your focus and concentration and provides a more thorough toning of your core, arms, and legs.

To perform this exercise, you must:

1. Part from the Plank Pose, pushing evenly through your hands and keeping your shoulders aligned over your wrists.

2. Steady your core and leg muscles, keeping them strong, and then roll both heels to the right, placing the outer edge of your right foot against the ground. Stack your left foot on top of the right.
3. Draw your legs in together and push out through your feet.
4. Inhale deeply and press down through your right hand, shifting your weight onto your right arm as you raise your left hand. Try to gaze at your raised hand if it's comfortable for your neck. If it's not comfortable, keep your head in a neutral position.
5. Firm your belly and lengthen your tailbone toward your heels.
6. Exhale and bring your thigh toward your chest, lifting your leg up toward the ceiling.
7. Hook your big toe with your fingers and secure the grip with your thumb.
8. Hold the pose for 30 seconds to a minute. Gradually increase your stay up to 2 minutes. Switch sides and repeat for the same length of time.

Scale Pose

Focus: Wrists; arms; abdomen
Level: Advanced
Sanskrit Name: *Tolasana*
Time: 10 to 20 seconds per side
Indications: Strengthening; improves balance
Contraindications: Ankle injuries; knee injuries; tight hips or thighs; shoulder injuries; wrist injuries

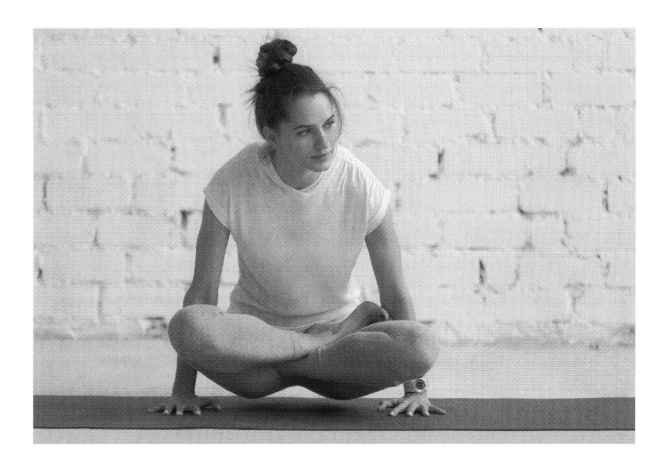

The Scale Pose is an advanced arm balance pose that strengthens your wrists, arms, and abs as you improve your sense of balance.

To perform this exercise, you must:

1. Part from the Lotus Pose and place your palms on the floor beside your hips.
2. Exhale and then prepare to push your hands against the floor, contracting your abdominal muscles and lifting your legs and buttocks away from the floor. If lifting your legs away from the floor is hard for you, try using a block underneath each hand to allow your arms to apply more strength and length to the push.
3. Hold the suspended pose for 10 to 20 seconds. Come up by lowering your legs and buttocks. Now change the cross of your legs and repeat the exercise on the other side for the same length of time.

Avoid this pose if you have any shoulder or wrist injury.

Yoga Poses for the Chest

Warrior Pose II

Focus: Chest; shoulders; legs; ankles
Level: Beginner
Sanskrit Name: *Virabhadrasana II*
Time: 30 seconds to a minute per side
Indications: Strengthening; stretching; abdominal stimulation
Contraindications: Diarrhea; neck injuries; high blood pressure

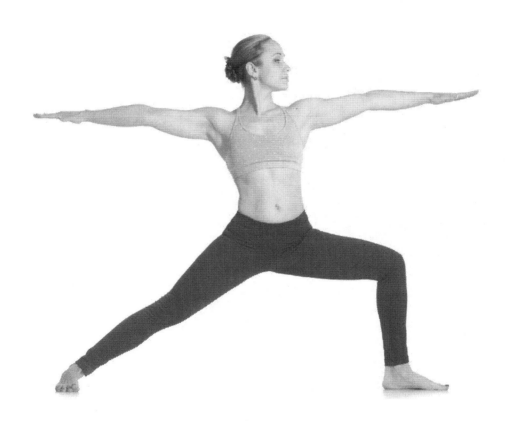

The Warrior Pose II is the follow-up of the Warrior Pose I, another of the three Warrior poses.

The effects of this pose don't differ too radically from the first. It stimulates the abdominal organs; stretches the groins, chest, lungs, and shoulders; and strengthens the legs and ankles.

Constant practice leads to increased stamina, and it's been reported as therapeutic for flat feet, sciatica, and osteoporosis.

1. Part from the Mountain Pose. Step your feet between 3-and-a-half to 4 feet apart.
2. Lift your arms parallel to the floor and reach them to the sides, shoulder blades wide, palms down.
3. Turn your right foot slightly to the right, about 45° to 60°, and your left foot out to the left about 90°. Make sure to align your heels.
4. Firm your thighs, turning your left thigh outward so as to keep your left kneecap in line with your left ankle.
5. Bend your left knee over your left ankle to keep the shin perpendicular to the floor. If you're flexible and strong enough, try keeping your left thigh parallel to the floor. Be sure to press your outer right heel firmly into the floor to anchor this movement.
6. Stretch your arms parallel to the floor. Try not to lean your torso over your left thigh. Both sides of your torso must remain equally long.
7. Stay between 30 seconds to a minute. Come up and repeat with your legs reversed for the same time.

Chair Pose

Focus: Chest; thighs; calves; ankles
Level: Beginner
Sanskrit Name: *Utkatasana*
Time: 30 seconds to a minute
Indications: Strengthening; stretching; opens chest
Contraindications: Headache; low blood pressure; insomnia

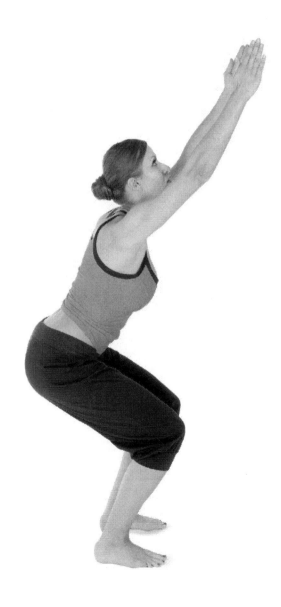

The Chair Pose is a great standing pose to open the chest and build up strength in the ankles, thighs, and calves.

To perform this exercise, you must:

1. Part from the Mountain Pose. Raise your arms perpendicular to the floor. Keep your arms parallel, facing inward, or your palms joined.
2. Exhale all the air you can from your lungs and then bend your knees. Position your thighs as parallel to the floor as you can.
3. Your knees should be ahead of your feet, and your torso should lean slightly over your thighs to form a right angle.
4. Press the heads of your thigh bones down to your heels to keep them parallel.
5. Firm your shoulder blades against your back and then send your tailbone down toward the floor.
6. To end this pose, straighten your knees as you inhale and lift through your arms.

30 seconds to a minute will be enough.

Half Frog Pose

Focus: Whole front body; ankles; thighs; groins; core; psoas
Level: Beginner-Intermediate
Sanskrit Name: *Ardha Bhekasana*
Time: At least 30 seconds, up to 2 minutes
Indications: Strengthening; stretching; opens chest; opens shoulders; improves pose
Contraindications: Low (or high) blood pressure; back injuries, neck injuries; shoulder injuries; migraine; insomnia

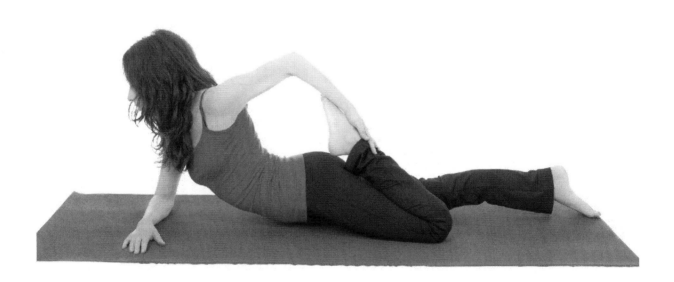

The Half-Frog Pose is a "beginner friendly" intermediate backbend pose that opens the chest, shoulders, and thighs just as it strengthens the back muscles and improves your pose.

To perform this exercise, you must:

1. Lie flat on your belly.
2. Press your forearms into the ground, lifting your head and upper torso as you do.
3. Bend your right knee and bring your right heel toward its buttock. Shifting your weight onto your left forearm, reach back with your right hand and grasp the inside of your right foot.
4. Slowly rotate your elbow toward the ceiling as you slide your fingers over the top of your foot, curling them over the toe tips. The base of your right palm should be pressing the top of the foot.
5. Press your foot toward the buttock. If you're flexible enough, take the foot slightly off to the side and push it down toward the floor. Its knee must remain in line with your hip, and you must make sure you're not pressing to the point your knee hurts.
6. Keep your shoulders squared and try not to fall into your left shoulder. To ensure this, press down with your elbow to lift your chest.
7. Hold the pose for 30 seconds, up to 2 minutes. End, take a few breaths, and perform the exercise again, on the other side, for the same time.

Lord of the Dance Pose

Focus: Shoulders; chest; thighs; groins; abdomen; legs; ankles
Level: Intermediate
Sanskrit Name: *Natarajasana*
Time: 20 to 30 seconds
Indications: Stretching; strengthening; improves balance
Contraindications: Ankle injuries; back injuries; low blood pressure

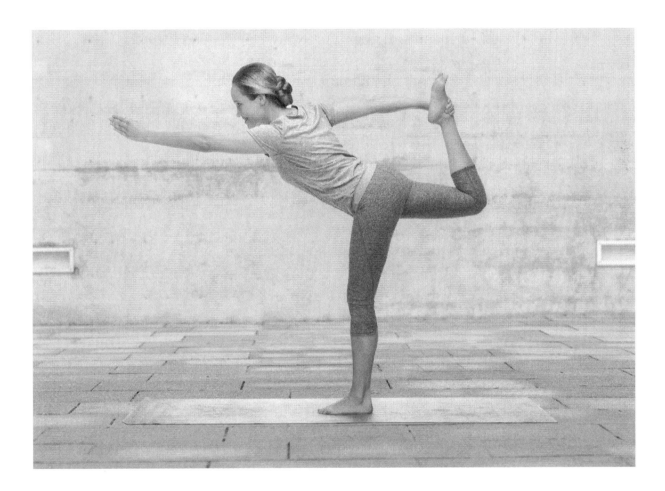

The Lord of the Dance Pose is a rigorous pose that demands equal parts of balance and strength. It strengthens the legs and ankles; stretches the shoulders, chest, thighs, groins, and abdomen; and improves the sense of balance.

To perform this exercise, you must:

1. Part from the Mountain Pose, shift your weight onto your right foot, and then lift your left heel toward your left buttock while you bend the knee.
2. Push back the head of your right thigh bone, deep into the hip joint, and then lift the kneecap to keep the standing leg stretched and balanced.
3. Keep your torso as upright as you can, and then either:
   a. Reach back with your left hand, grasping the outside of your left foot or ankle. To avoid compressing your lower back, lift your pubis toward your navel as you push your tailbone toward the floor. Lift your left foot off the floor and back from your torso, then extend your left thigh behind you and turn it parallel to the floor. Extend your right arm forward in front your torso, keeping it parallel to the floor.
   b. Sweep your right hand around and behind your back, and then grasp your inner left foot. Sweep your left hand back and grasp the outside of your left foot. Now extend your left thigh behind you and keep it parallel to the floor. This option demands more balance.
4. Regardless of your choice, hold the pose between 20 and 30 seconds. End by releasing your grasp on your foot, and then repeat for the same time on the other side.

Beginners should pay attention to the back of their thighs. If you don't keep the ankle of the raised foot flexed, you might end up cramping the back of the thigh. Drawing the top of the foot toward the shin will help you keep the ankle flexed.

Extended Side Angle Pose

Focus: Groins; spine; waist; chest; shoulders; legs; knees; ankles
Level: Intermediate
Sanskrit Name: *Utthita Parsvakonasana*
Time: 30 seconds to a minute per side
Indications: Stretching; strengthening; abdominal stimulation
Contraindications: Headache; low (or high) blood pressure; insomnia

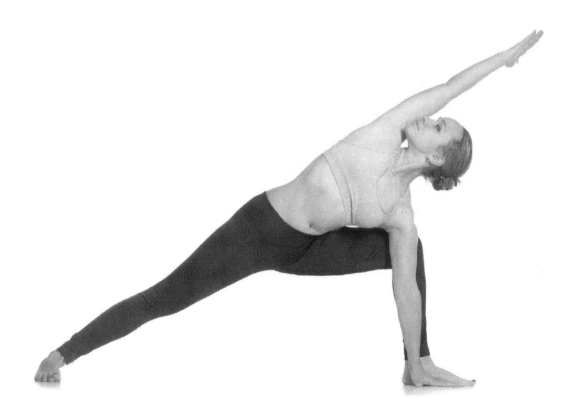

The Extended Side Angle Pose is a twist pose that stretches the groins, spine, waist, chest, and shoulders as it strengthens the knees, legs, and ankles.

To perform this exercise, you must:

1. Part from the Mountain Pose and then separate your feet 3-and-a-half to 4 feet apart.
2. Extend your arms, keeping them parallel to the floor, and swing them to the sides, palms down.

3. Turn your left foot slightly to the right and your right foot all the way to the right (90°). Align both heels.
4. Firm your thighs and turn your right thigh outward, keeping the kneecap in line with the center of your right ankle.
5. Move your left hip slightly forward to the right as you rotate your upper torso back to the left.
6. Move your inner left groin deep into the pelvis to anchor your left heel into the floor.
7. Bend your right knee over your right ankle, keeping your shin perpendicular to the floor. If possible, bring your right thigh parallel to the floor.
8. Firm your shoulder blades against your back ribs. Extend your left arm toward the ceiling, and turn your left palm to face your head. Reach the arm over the back of your left ear.
9. Lengthen the entire left side of your body by stretching from your left heel to your left fingertips.
10. Turn your head to look at your left arm, and release your right shoulder away from the ear. Keep the length along the right side of your torso equal to the length along the left side.
11. Ground your left heel to the floor as you lay the right side of your torso onto the top of your right thigh. Bring it as close as you can. Push your right palm into the floor outside your right foot, and then press your right knee back against the inner arm as you burrow your tailbone into the back of your pelvis. Your inner right thigh should be parallel with the ground.
12. Hold the pose for 30 seconds to a minute. Inhale and press your heels into the ground, then reach your left arm toward the ceiling to lighten the movement. Take a few breaths and then repeat the exercise but reversed.

Revolved Side Angle Pose

Focus: Groins; spine; waist; chest; shoulders; legs; knees; ankles
Level: Intermediate
Sanskrit Name: *Parivrtta Parsvakonasana*
Time: 30 seconds to a minute per side
Indications: Stretching; strengthening; abdominal stimulation; improves balance
Contraindications: Headache; low (or high) blood pressure; insomnia

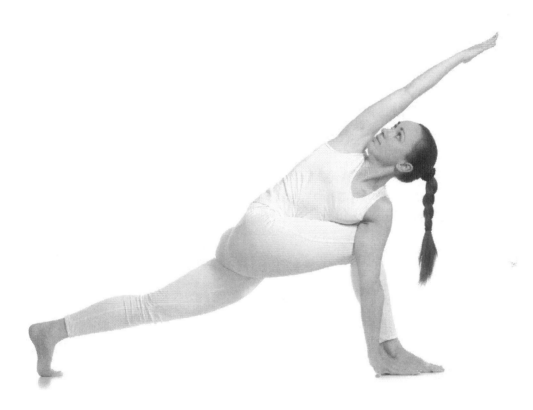

The Revolved Side Angle Pose is a revolved, harder variation of the Extended Side Angle Pose that will demand more flexibility and endurance.

It stretches the groins, spine, chest, and shoulders; strengthens the legs, knees, and ankles; and improves balance.

To perform this exercise, you must:

1. Part from the Mountain Pose. Separate your feet 3-and-a-half to 4 feet apart and rest your hands on your hips. Turn your left foot slightly to the right, and turn your right foot to the right 90°. Align both heels.
2. Firm your thighs and turn your right thigh out so that the kneecap is centered with the ankle.
3. Turn your torso to the right until you're directly facing your right leg. Lift your left heel from the floor and spin it until your inner left foot is parallel to your inner right foot.
4. Bend your right knee, if possible, until your right thigh is parallel to the floor. Press your left thigh up and extend through your left heel. To resist the lift, press your tailbone toward your pubis.
5. Turn further to the right and bend your torso down, resting your left hand on the floor beside your inner right foot. Sink your right thumb into your right hip crease and push the thighbone down to the ground.
6. Firm your shoulder blades into your back ribs and lift your torso back slightly for a few breaths. What comes after might be more challenging. If you're having problems at this point, skip to the last step.
7. Bend your left elbow and move it to the outside of your right knee. Nestle the knee and elbow against each other. If you can, straighten your left elbow and extend your hand toward the ground. (If you can't, use a support like a block or a bolster.)
8. Keep your right hand on your hip or stretch it over the back of your right ear. Then turn your head to look at your right arm. (Don't do this if you've got any sort of neck problems; in that case, just keep your head in a neutral position looking down at the ground.)
9. Hold the pose for at least half a minute, but gradually increase your stay up to a minute. When you're ready to come up, take a few breaths, and then reverse your feet and repeat.

Wild Thing Pose

Focus: Chest; shoulders; legs; psoas; back
Level: Intermediate
Sanskrit Name: *Camatkarasana*
Time: 30 seconds to a minute per side
Indications: Stretching; strengthening; opens chest
Contraindications: Wrist injuries; carpal tunnel syndrome

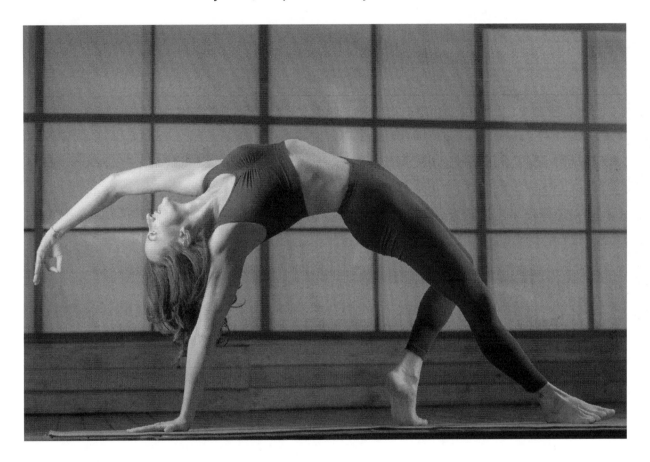

The Wild Thing Pose is a beginner-intermediate pose that opens the chest, lung, and shoulders; stretches the legs and psoas; and strengthens the shoulders and upper back.

To perform this exercise, you must:

1. Part from the Downward Facing Dog Pose, and then shift your weight to your right hand.
2. Roll onto the outer edge of your right foot, just like you do in the Side Plank Pose.

3. Lift your hips with buoyancy and strengthen your right hand. Exhalation after exhalation, work your left foot back and rest your toes on the ground, partially bending your knee.
4. Curl back your upper back to swing your shoulder blades into the back of your rib cage.
5. Breathe easily, curling your head back as you do. Extend your left arm from your heart in a symbolic display of power and freedom.
6. Hold the pose for any length of time between the span of 5 to 10 breaths, and then step back into the Downward Facing Dog Pose and repeat the pose on the other side.

Camel Pose

Focus: Whole front body; ankles; thighs; groins; psoas; back
Level: Beginner
Sanskrit Name: *Ustrasana*
Time: Up to a minute
Indications: Strengthening; stretching; opens chest; abdominal stimulation
Contraindications: Back injuries; insomnia; migraine; neck injuries; low (or high) blood pressure

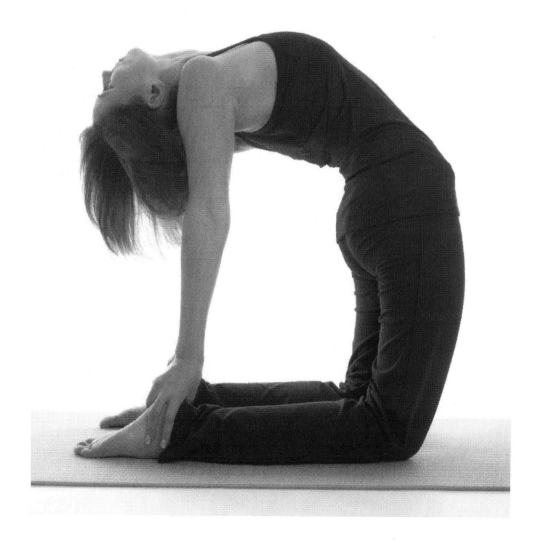

The Camel Pose is a challenging seated chest opener pose that will stretch almost all your body. It will also strengthen your back muscles and stimulate your abdominal organs.

To perform this exercise, you must:

1. Kneel on the floor, knees hip-width apart and thighs perpendicular to the floor.
2. Firm your buttocks and keep your outer hips as soft as possible.
3. Press your shins and the tops of your feet evenly against the floor.
4. Place your hands on the back of your pelvis, laying them on top of your buttocks, and use them to spread your pelvis. To keep your front groins from puffing forward, press your front thighs back.
5. Press your shoulder blades against your ribs to bring your heart up.
6. Lean back against your tailbone and shoulder blades. Keep your hands on your pelvis and your head up.
7. Press your palms into your soles or heels. Your fingers should point toward your toes.
8. You should turn your arms so that your elbow creases face forward, but don't squeeze your shoulder blades together. You can keep your neck neutral or dropped in the back; in any case, be extra careful not to strain it.
9. End the pose by bringing your hands to the front of your pelvis, and then lifting your head and torso up by pushing your hip points down.

This pose is naturally difficult for the neck, and it can lead to serious strain and injury, especially for beginners. To prepare for this, you can use a wall to press the crown of your head into. Don't spend more than a minute like this.

King Cobra Pose

Focus: Spine; chest; shoulders; back
Level: Intermediate
Sanskrit Name: *Raja Bhujangasana*
Time: 30 seconds to a minute and a half
Indications: Stretching; strengthening; opens chest
Contraindications: Ankle injuries; knee injuries; back injuries

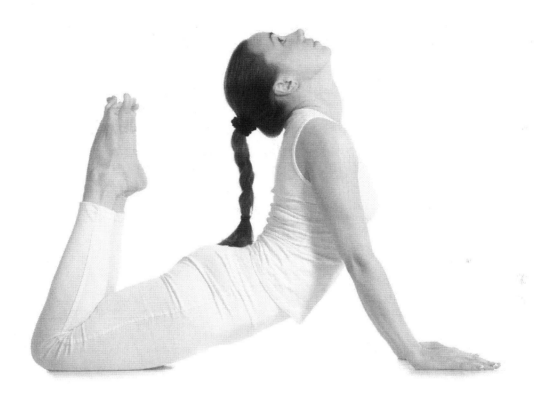

The King Cobra Pose is a tougher variation of the Cobra Pose which exacts a more demanding bend in the spine.

It thoroughly stretches the spine; opens the chest and shoulders; invigorates the energy; and strengthens all the muscles in the back.

To perform this exercise, you must:

1. Lie prone on the floor, belly down. Rest your forehead on the floor.
2. Locate your hands beneath your shoulders, spreading your palms on the ground.
3. Drag your shoulders blades down toward your hips while you nestle your elbows nicely into your ribs.
4. Push firmly into the ground with the tops of your feet and pubic bone.
5. Inhale, and then lift your head forward as you lift your chest off the ground to enter the Cobra Pose.
6. Engage the abdominals, sending your navel in toward your spine, protecting your lower back. Push through your hands, and use your back muscles to lift further toward the ceiling. Extend your arms.
7. Try spreading your legs so that your knees extend as much as they can. Lift your torso off the floor as much as possible.
8. Reach your head up and bend into your neck.
9. Bend your knees, bringing your toes toward your head.
10. Hold the pose for 30 seconds to a minute. Work your stay up to a minute and a half, take a few breaths, and then slowly lower your body into the floor.

Noose Pose

Focus: Ankles; thighs; groins; spine; chest; shoulders
Level: Advanced
Sanskrit Name: *Pasasana*
Time: 30 seconds to 1 minute per side
Indications: Stretching; strengthening; opens chest; abdominal stimulation
Contraindications: Knee injuries; back injuries; disk hernias

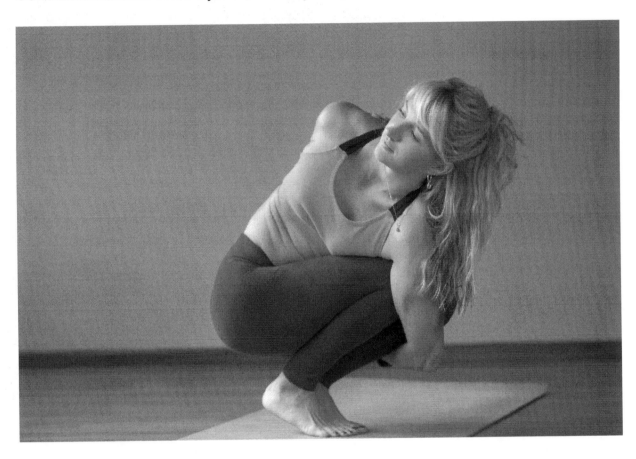

The Noose Pose is a challenging pose that stretches and strengthens the ankles, thighs, groins, and spine; opens the chest and shoulders; and stimulates the belly organs.

To perform this exercise, you must:

1. Part from the Mountain Pose, with a wall next to your right side, keeping your feet hip-width and parallel to each other.
2. Turn to the right, pressing your right palm into the wall from wrist to elbow, with your forearm parallel to the ground.

3. Bend your knees into a full squat, resting your buttocks on top of your heels. If you can't fully ground your heels, slide a folded blanket underneath.
4. Swing your knees gently to the left, exhale, and then turn your torso to the right, pressing both hands into the wall. As your left hand pushes the wall, your elbow should hug the outside of your right knee.
5. For the pose to work, you must close any space between the left side of your torso and the tops of your thighs. A good way of going about this is working the back of your left arm down your leg, moving your left shoulder toward the outside of your right knee.
6. Press your knee and arm evenly against each other and use this pressure to lengthen the left side of your torso beyond the inner groins, swaying along the top of the thighs. The trick lies in keeping your belly as soft as possible.
7. You can keep your right hand on the wall, but you should gradually get to the point where you clasp your palms together, elbows angled away from each other, using the pressure of your grip to boost the twist.
8. Hold this pose for 30 seconds to a minute, then release gently and repeat on the other side.

One-Legged King Pigeon Pose I

Focus: Thighs; groins; chest; shoulders; psoas; abdomen
Level: Advanced
Sanskrit Name: *Eka Pada Rajakapotasana I*
Time: 30 seconds to a minute per side
Indications: Stretching; abdominal stimulation; opens chest
Contraindications: Sacroiliac injuries; ankle injuries; knee injuries; tight hips or thighs

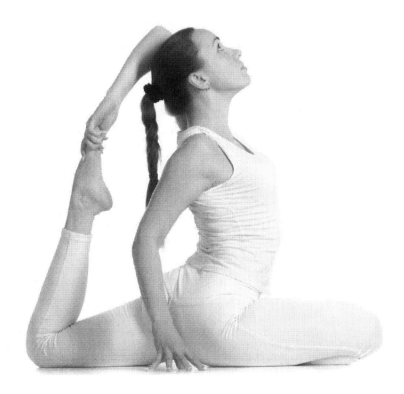

The One-Legged King Pigeon Pose I is a variation of the advanced backbend King Pigeon pose. It strongly stretches the thighs, groins, psoas, chest, shoulders, and abs; stimulates the belly organs; and puffs the chest.

To perform this exercise, you must:

1. Get on the floor on all fours, placing your legs directly below your hips, with your hands just a bit ahead of your shoulders.
2. Slide your right knee forward, to the back of your right wrist, while you angle your right shin under your torso.
3. Move your right foot toward the front of your left knee. The outside of your right shin should rest comfortably on the ground.
4. Slide your left leg back, straightening the knee to descend the front of the thigh to the floor.
5. Push the outside of your right buttock to the floor, and then place your right heel just in front of the left hip.
6. You can angle your right knee slightly to the right, outside the line of the hip. Look back at your left leg; it should extend straight out of the hip, without being angled off to the left. Rotate it slightly to the inside, so that the midline presses against the floor.
7. Lay your torso down on top of your inner right thigh for a few breaths. Exhale and then stretch your arms forward.
8. Slide your hands back toward your front shin, and then press your fingers firmly into the floor to lift your torso away from your thigh.
9. Press your tailbone down and forward to lengthen your lower back while lifting your pubis toward the navel.
10. Roll your left hip point toward your right heel, and then lengthen your left front groin.
11. Try to maintain the upright position of your hands on the floor, then bring your hands to the top rim of your pelvis. Press down, and with the pressure, lift the lower rim of your rib cage.
12. Without compressing your neck, drop your head back, and then lift your chest by pushing the top of your sternum (at the manubrium) toward the ceiling.
13. Hold the pose for a minute or so. End by sliding your left knee forward, and then step back into the Downward Facing Dog Pose. Take a couple of breaths, and then repeat the pose with your legs reversed.

One-Legged King Pigeon Pose II

Focus: Thighs; groins; chest; shoulders; psoas; abdomen
Level: Advanced
Sanskrit Name: *Eka Pada Rajakapotasana II*
Time: 15 to 30 seconds per side
Indications: Stretching; strengthening; abdominal stimulation; improves pose
Contraindications: Low (or high) blood pressure; migraine; insomnia; back injuries; neck injuries

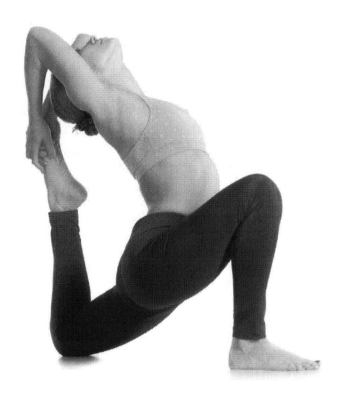

The One-Legged King Pigeon Pose II is the second variation of the advanced backbend King Pigeon pose.

Like its parent, it allows you to stretch the entire front body, strengthens the hip flexors and back, improves pose, and stimulates the abdominal organs.

To perform this exercise, you must:

1. Part from the Staff Pose and bend your right knee, placing your foot flat on the floor in front of your right sit bone. Your shin should be somewhat perpendicular to the ground.
2. Lean slightly to the right and swing your left leg straight back behind your torso. Place it, fully extended, on the floor, keeping the top of the foot on the floor.
3. Now bend your left knee and raise your shin somewhat perpendicular to the floor. Your body weight should balance on your right foot and left knee (if you're flexible, try balancing on your thigh as well). Secure your position by pushing your right knee forward until it sticks out slightly beyond your right toes.
4. Lift your right arm up, bend your elbow, and take the left foot. Do the same with your left arm.
5. Clasp your foot firmly, lift your chest, and then drop your head back, toward the sole of your left foot. Push your elbows toward the ceiling.
6. Hold the pose for 15 to 30 seconds, breathing as easily as you can. Come down by exhaling as you release your left foot, bringing the leg back to the floor. Take a few breaths, and then repeat the exercise on the other side for the same amount of time.

Yoga Poses for the Back

Crocodile Pose

Focus: Spine; back
Level: Beginner
Sanskrit Name: *Makarasana*
Time: At least a minute
Indications: Body relaxation; mental relaxation
Contraindications: Mid- to late-term pregnancy

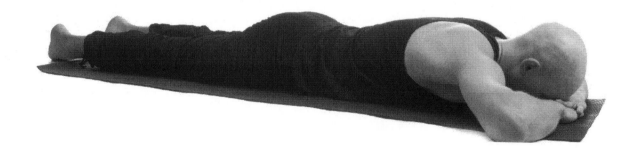

The Crocodile Pose is a restorative pose that relieves tension from the spine and back; regulates blood pressure; soothes the mind; and reduces anxiety.

To perform this exercise, you must:

1. Lie prone on the ground, belly down. Cross both arms under your head.
2. Rest your forehead on your wrists and close your eyes; let your whole body relax, sinking into the floor. Let your heels turn out, and let your legs flop open.
3. Breathe deeply and evenly. Push your belly down into the floor with each inhale, and maintain this action for 6 to 10 breaths. Each exhalation should release tension from your body down into the Earth.
4. Come up by bringing your palms under your shoulders to lift your chest. The Child Pose is a usual follow-up for this pose.

Cobra Pose

Focus: Chest; spine
Level: Beginner
Sanskrit Name: *Bhujangasana*
Time: 15 to 30 seconds
Indications: Strengthening; stretching; opens the chest; abdominal stimulation
Contraindications: Pregnancy; headache; back injuries; carpal tunnel syndrome

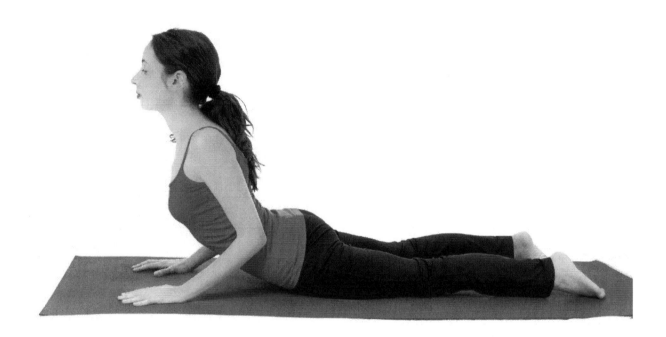

The Cobra Pose is an excellent backbend pose to open the chest, strengthen the spine, and stimulate the abdominal organs, heart, and lungs.

If your floor is not comfortable, I recommend rolling out a folded blanket to soften the surface. Pregnant women and those with back injuries should avoid this pose.

To perform this exercise, you must:

1. Lie prone on the ground. Stretch your legs back, placing the tops of your feet on the floor. Spread your hands just in front of your shoulders. Place your elbows against your body.
2. Press your thighs, the tops of your feet, and your pubis firmly against the floor.
3. Inhale and then straighten your arms, lifting your chest off the floor. Go as far up as you can while keeping your pubis connected to your legs.
4. Firm your shoulder blades in your back, puffing your side ribs forward. You should distribute the backbend evenly throughout your spine.
5. Hold the pose while breathing easily for 15 to 30 seconds.

If you're more flexible, you could push your hands a little farther, straighten your elbows, and lift the top of your sternum to move into a deeper backbend.

Marichi Pose

Focus: Spine; shoulders; hips
Level: Beginner
Sanskrit Name: *Marichyasana III*
Time: 30 seconds to a minute
Indications: Strengthening; stretching; mental relaxation; abdominal stimulation
Contraindications: Diarrhea; insomnia; headache or migraine; low (or high) blood pressure

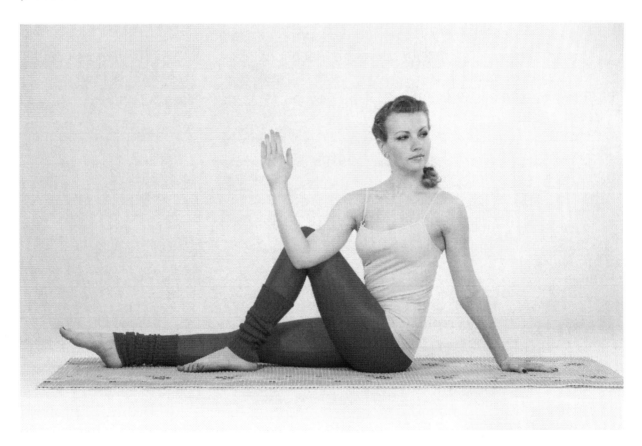

The Marichi Pose is a twisting yoga pose that stretches the shoulders; massages the belly organs; eases hip pain; and strengthens the spine.

To perform this exercise, you must:

1. Part from the Staff Pose. Bend your right knee in and rest your sole on the floor, keeping the heel as close as you can to your right sit bone. Your left leg should be kept strong and rotated slightly to the inside.

2. Ground the head of the thigh bone into the floor. Push the back of your left heel and the base of the big toe off the pelvis. Press the right foot into the floor, softening the inner right groin to receive the pubis in the twist.
3. Ground the thigh of the stretched leg and bent-knee foot to lengthen your spine.
4. Rotate your torso to the right as you exhale, wrapping your left arm around the right thigh. Hold the outmost part with your left hand, pulling the thigh up as you release the right hip into the floor.
5. Push your right hand onto the floor behind your pelvis to lift your torso up and forward.
6. Drag your inner right groin deep into the pelvis, and lengthen your front belly up out of the groin in line with your inner right thigh.
7. Keep lengthening your spine with each inhalation, twisting a little more with each exhalation.
8. Hug the thigh to your belly while you lean your back into your shoulder blades.
9. Turn your head to the right to twist in your cervical spine.
10. Hold the pose for 30 seconds to a minute.

Seated Forward Bend

Focus: Spine; shoulders; hamstrings; back
Level: Beginner
Sanskrit Name: *Paschimottanasana*
Time: 1 to 3 minutes
Indications: Stretching; abdominal stimulation; mental relaxation; improves digestion
Contraindications: Diarrhea; asthma; back injuries; late-term pregnancy

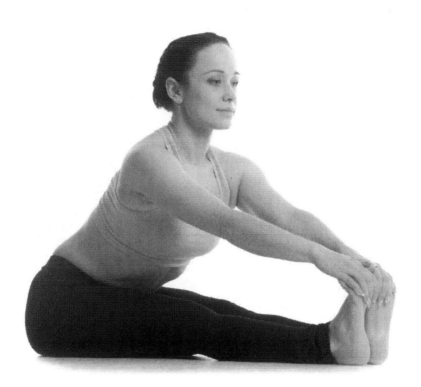

The seated forward bend is a beginner forward bend pose that stretches the spine, shoulders, and hamstrings. It's perfect for novice yogis and it can be very mentally stimulating.

I recommend rolling a folded blanket out on the ground.

To perform this exercise, you must:

1. Sit on the floor, supporting your buttocks on a folded blanket. Stretch your legs in front of you. Press firmly through your heels. Sway a little onto your left buttock to recoil your right sit bone away from the heel with your right hand. Do the same on the other side.
2. Turn your thighs slightly to the inside, then press them down into the ground.
3. Push your hands against the floor beside your hips to lift your sternum toward the ceiling while dropping your top thighs lower.
4. Drag your groins into your pelvis. Keep your front torso long, leaning forward from your hip joints.
5. Lengthen your tailbone away from the back of your pelvis and try to clasp the sides of your feet with your hands. If that's not possible for you, loop a strap around the soles of your feet, hold it firmly, and walk it gently as much as you can while keeping your elbows straight.
6. As you lengthen your front torso, keep your arms long and your elbows out to the sides. Your lower belly should touch your thighs first; then continue all the way up to your head.
7. Hold the pose for 1 to 3 minutes. Come up gently by lifting your torso away from your thighs.

Extended Puppy Pose

Focus: Spine; shoulders
Level: Beginner
Sanskrit Name: *Uttana Shishosana*
Time: 30 seconds to 1 minute
Indications: Stretching; mental relaxation
Contraindications: Knee injuries

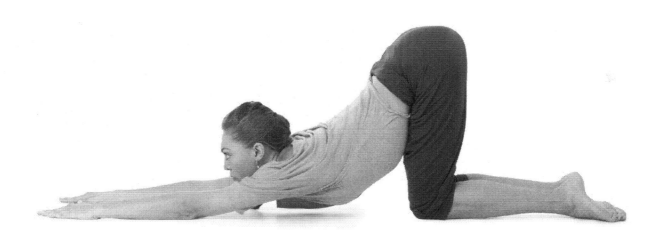

The Extended Puppy Pose is a combination of the Child's Pose and the Downward Facing Dog Pose. It stretches the spine and shoulders and soothes the mind.

To perform this exercise, you must:

1. Get down on the floor on all fours. Ensure that your shoulders are above your wrists and your hips are above your knees.
2. Move your hands forward, just a few inches, and curl your toes under.
3. Move your buttocks halfway back toward your heels as you exhale. Try to keep your arms active, without your elbows touching the ground.

4. Drop your forehead to the floor. If this isn't too comfortable, slide a folded blanket underneath.
5. Keep your lower back slightly compressed and press your hands down, stretching through your arms as you pull your hips back toward your heels.
6. Breathe into your back, lengthening your spine in both directions.
7. Hold the pose for 30 seconds to a minute. Take a few breaths, and then release your buttocks down onto your heels.

Consider sliding some folded blankets below your knees to protect them.

Knee Press Pose

Focus: Back; belly; abdomen; legs; arms
Level: Beginner
Sanskrit Name: *Pavanamuktasana*
Time: At least 20 seconds in each stage
Indications: Stretching; strengthening; abdominal stimulation; improves digestion
Contraindications: Hernias; spine injuries; sciatica; pregnancy

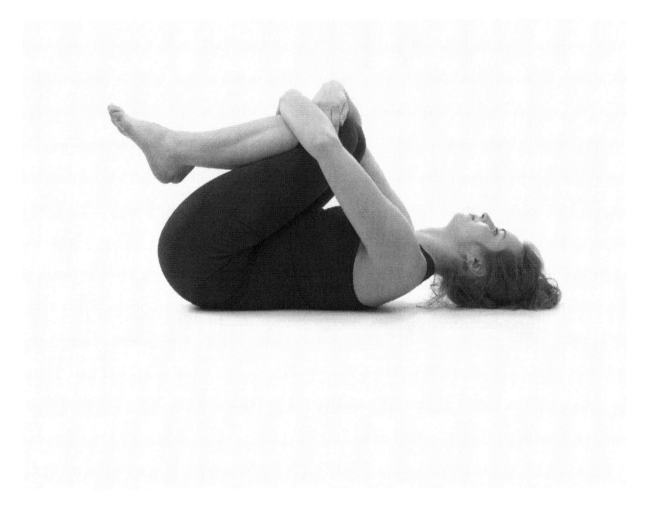

The Knee Press Pose is a restorative pose that strengthens the back and abdominal muscles; tones the belly, legs, and arms; eases tension from the lower back; and—most importantly—massages the digestive organs (such as the intestines), helping the release of gasses.

To perform this exercise, you must:

1. Lie supine on your back, keeping your feet together and your arms beside your torso.
2. Bend your right leg toward your torso, clasp your thigh with both hands, and press it down to your abdomen.
3. Breathe in, lift your head and chest off the floor, and try to touch your right knee with your chin.
4. Hold it for a few breaths, and then straighten your leg back onto the floor.
5. Repeat the exercise with the other leg.
6. Now do the exercise with both legs, clasping each thigh with each hand.
7. Try rolling side to side, 3 to 5 times, and then take a few breaths to release.

Boat Pose

Focus: Abdomen; psoas; spine
Level: Intermediate
Sanskrit Name: *Paripurna Navasana*
Time: 10 seconds, up to a minute
Indications: Strengthening; toning; abdominal stimulation
Contraindications: Asthma; diarrhea; headache; heart problems; low blood pressure; insomnia; neck injury; mid- to late-term pregnancy

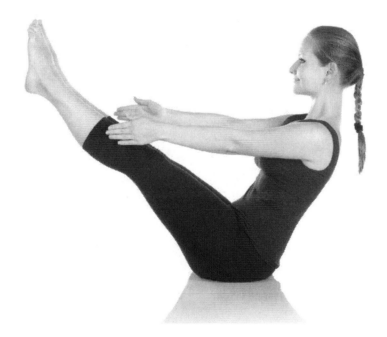

The Boat Pose is a deep hip flexor strengthening pose that tones the abs; strengthens the psoas and spine; and stimulates the abdominal organs.

To perform this exercise, you must:

1. Sit on the floor, stretching your legs in front of you. Push your hands into the floor behind and slightly away from your hips; your fingers should point toward your feet.

2. Lift through the top of your sternum, leaning back slightly as you do. Make sure you don't compress your back.
3. Lengthen the front of your torso between the pubis and top sternum. Sit on your two sitting bones and tailbone to form the "tripod" with which this pose stands.
4. Bend your knees and then lift your feet off the ground. Your thighs should be angled about 45° to 50° relative to the floor. Continue to lengthen your tailbone into the floor and raise your pubis toward your navel. Try to slowly straighten your knees and raise the tips of your toes slightly above the level of your eyes. If you can't keep your knees straight, keep them bent and lift your shins so that they're parallel to the floor.
5. Stretch your arms beside your legs, keeping them parallel to each other and the floor. Widen your shoulder blades across your back. If you can't, keep your hands on the floor beside your hips, or grasp the backs of your thighs.
6. Your lower belly should be firm, not hard or thick. Try to keep it relatively flat.
7. Push the heads of your thigh bones toward the floor to help anchor the pose and lift your top sternum. Tip your chin toward your sternum to lift the base of your skull away from the back of your neck. Breathe easily.
8. Initially, holding the pose for 10–20 seconds will be enough, but gradually increase the time of your stay to a minute. Release your legs as you exhale and then sit on an inhalation.

If straightening your legs becomes difficult, try bending your knees and looping a strap around the soles of your feet. Grip the strap firmly and then lean your torso back, adjust the strap to keep it taut, and push your feet firmly against the strap.

Head to Knee Forward Bend Pose

Focus: Spine; back; shoulders; hamstrings; groins
Level: Beginner
Sanskrit Name: *Janu Sirsasana*
Time: 1 to 3 minutes per side
Indications: Stretching; strengthening; stimulation; mental relaxation
Contraindications: Diarrhea; asthma; knee injuries; late-term pregnancy

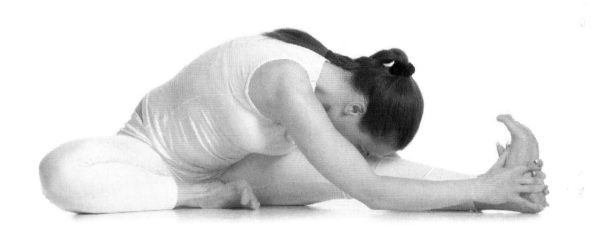

The Head to Knee Forward Bend Pose is a powerful forward bend that stretches the spine, back, shoulders, hamstrings, and groins; stimulates the abdominal organs; and calms the brain.

Yogis seeking to strengthen their spines should master this pose.

To perform this exercise, you must:

1. Sit on the floor, legs stretched in front of you. Bend your right knee, drawing the heel back to your perineum.

2. Rest your right sole gently against your inner left thigh. Lay your outer right leg on the floor, keeping the shin at a right angle with your left leg. If your right knee doesn't sit comfortably, roll a folded blanket below.
3. Push your right hand against your inner right groin, where the pelvis joins the thigh. Press your left hand on the ground beside your hip. Gently turn your torso to the left, lifting it as you ground your inner right thigh.
4. Align your navel with the center of your left thigh.
5. You can loop a strap to your left foot and walk your right hand along the strap to lengthen your spine evenly. Alternatively, reach out with your right hand, clasping your left foot with your thumb on the sole.
6. Use your left hand to push yourself over to increase the pressure of the twist. Then reach your left foot with your left hand.
7. Lengthen your front torso from the pubis to the sternum. Ideally, you shouldn't place too much force in the pull. Bend your elbows out to the sides as you take them off the floor.
8. Keep lengthening forward until your lower belly touches your thighs.
9. Hold the pose for 1 to 3 minutes. Come up gently, take a few breaths, and repeat the instructions with the legs reversed.

Happy Baby Pose

Focus: Inner groins; spine
Level: Beginner
Sanskrit Name: *Ananda Balasana*
Time: At least a minute, up to 3
Indications: Stretching; mental relaxation
Contraindications: Mid- to late-term pregnancy; knee injuries; neck injuries

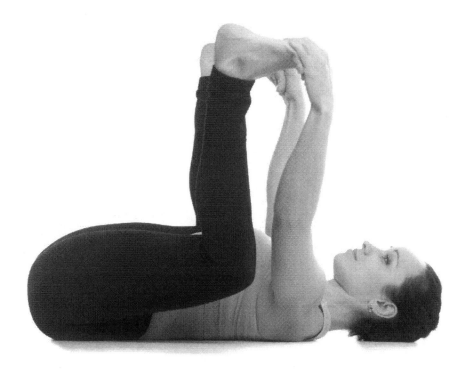

The Happy Baby Pose is a powerful inner groin and back stretching pose that will help relieve stress and fatigue.

To perform this exercise, you must:

1. Lie down on the floor on your back. Gently bend your knees into your belly.
2. Grip the outsides of your feet with your hands. Separate your knees from each other just slightly wider than your torso, and then bring them up toward your armpits.

3. Each ankle should be directly over the knee. Push your feet up into your hands while you pull them down to generate resistance. Apply just a little force.
4. To end the pose, let go of your feet and slowly bring your knees down, planting your feet firmly on the floor.

This pose is excellent when you've been working on the computer for hours. If you have some issues holding your feet initially, don't fret! Use a belt or a similar object looped over your soles and grab onto it instead.

Following up with the Downward Facing Dog Pose can do wonders for your entire body!

Hold the pose for at least a minute. Gradually build your endurance up to 3 minutes. Try to take 3 to 7 even breaths before ending, unless you feel too uncomfortable.

Warrior Pose III

Focus: Ankles; legs; shoulders; back; abdomen
Level: Intermediate
Sanskrit Name: *Virabhadrasana III*
Time: 30 to 40 seconds per side
Indications: Strengthening; toning; improves balance; improves pose
Contraindications: High blood pressure; ankle injuries

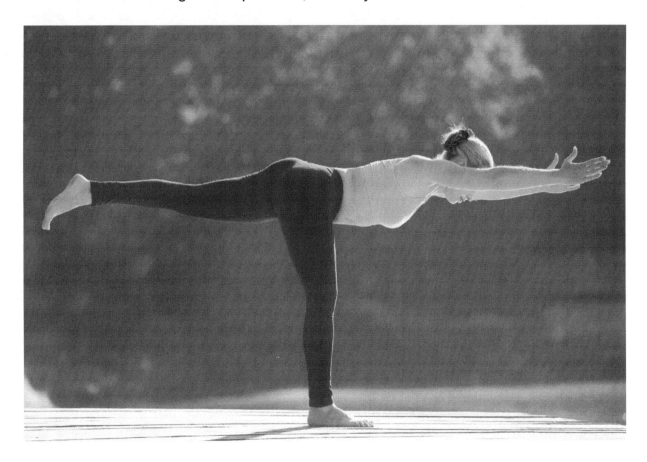

The Warrior Pose III is the third and last pose of the three Warrior Poses.
This pose will prove challenging to master. Nonetheless, the prospective yogi must strive to control it.

This asana will improve balance and pose, tone the abdomen, and strengthen the ankles, legs, shoulders, and back.

To perform this exercise, you must:

1. Part from the Mountain Pose. Fold forward to the Standing Forward Bend Pose and then step your left foot back into a high lunge position.
2. Lay the midline of your torso (pubis to sternum) down the midline of your right thigh (knee to hip crease) and then bring your hands to your right knee, clasping the inner and outer parts with the right and left hand respectively.
3. Lift your torso slightly, and turn it slightly to the right while squeezing the knee with your hands.
4. From this position, stretch your arms forward, parallel to the floor and each other, palms facing each other.
5. Press the head of your right thighbone back and press the heel actively into the floor. Straighten the front leg as you lift the back leg. Resist by pressing your tailbone into the pelvis.
6. Firmly ground your heels into the floor, allowing you to stabilize your position. Lunging your torso forward might destabilize you.
7. Your arms, torso, and raised leg should be somewhat parallel to the floor. The trick to remain both balanced and parallel is reaching out with your legs as far and strong as you can, while reaching forward with your arms just as much. Releasing the hip of the raised leg toward the floor will help as well.
8. You *should* stay in this position for as long as a minute, but 30 or 40 seconds will suffice. Take deep, even breaths as you do to remain balanced and focused.
9. Once you're ready, bring your hands to the floor beside your right foot. Step your left foot forward, take a breath, and then repeat the exercise on the other leg for the same amount of time.

With this we conclude the warrior poses. The most advanced students can progress from the Warrior Pose I to the Warrior Pose III by leaning forward, arms extended, while raising and extending their back leg.

Mastering the warrior poses will take you some time; there's no need to rush it. A partner or teacher will make the process much easier.

Plow Pose

Focus: Shoulders; spine
Level: Intermediate
Sanskrit Name: *Halasana*
Time: 1 to 5 minutes
Indications: Stretching; mental relaxation; abdominal stimulation
Contraindications: Diarrhea; asthma; high blood pressure; pregnancy; neck injuries

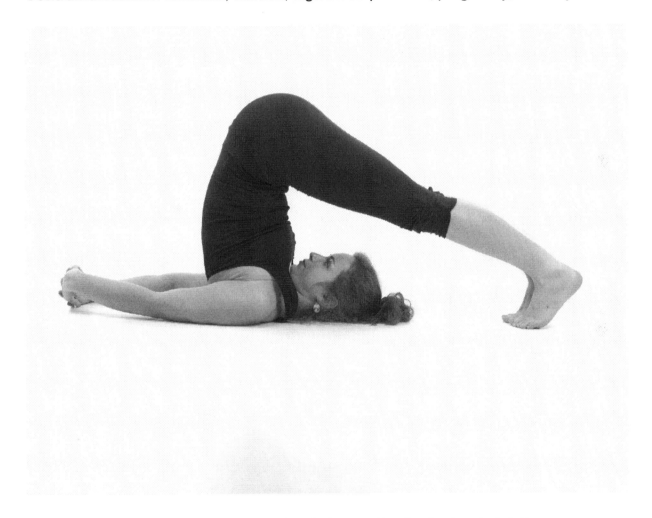

The Plow Pose is a stimulating pose that helps soothe the brain, stretch the shoulders and spine, and reduce stress. It can also help alleviate backache!

This pose is aimed at the intermediate–advanced yogi. It should be practiced with care, and after you can perform the Supported Shoulderstand Pose.

To perform this exercise, you must:

1. Part from the Supported Shoulderstand Pose and bend your hips from the joints to slowly lower your toes to the floor beyond your head. Keep your torso as perpendicular as you can.
2. With your legs as extended as possible, lift your top thighs and tailbone toward the ceiling and drag your inner groins deep into your pelvis. Continue to lift your chin away from your sternum.
3. Push your hand against the back of your torso to lift your back up toward the ceiling. Alternatively, you can release your hands away from your back and stretch your arms out behind you on the floor, opposite to the legs.
4. Clasp your hands together and then press down your arms on your support to lift your thighs toward the ceiling.
5. You should hold the pose between 1 and 5 minutes. To come up, bring your hands onto your back again, lifting yourself into the Supported Shoulderstand Pose again, and then roll down onto your back.

Beginners often overstretch their necks because they drag the shoulder blades far from the ears. To avoid this, firm your shoulder blades against your back to open your sternum.

If resting your feet on the floor isn't comfortable/possible for you, placing a block to rest your feet on is a solution. Not only does it help you achieve the same balance, it's better for your neck.

Frog Pose

Focus: Legs; spine; shoulders; groins
Level: Advanced
Sanskrit Name: *Bhekasana*
Time: At least 30 seconds, up to 2 minutes
Indications: Stretching; improves digestion; abdominal stimulation
Contraindications: Ankle injuries; back injuries; shoulder injuries; low blood pressure

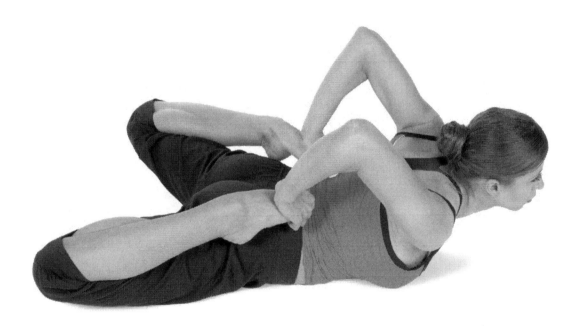

The Frog Pose is an intense leg stretch pose that can help improve and clean the digestive organs; stretch the whole legs, groins, spine, and shoulders; and stimulate the abdominal organs.

To perform this exercise, you must:

1. Sit on the floor. Keep your legs crossed and your body loosened.
2. Bring your hands behind you, lifting your chest in the process. Let your collarbones widen and lengthen your neck.

3. Lie upside-down, shifting your weight on your belly. Keep your feet hip-width apart, and slowly raise them up and back towards your buttocks with your toes pointing toward the ceiling.

4. Stretch your arms behind you and clasp both your feet with your hands. Squeeze your shoulders together and keep lifting your chest. The higher it is, the easier it becomes to hold your feet.

5. Hold this pose for 30 seconds to a minute. Gradually increase your stay up to 2 minutes.

Lotus Shoulderstand Pose

Focus: Back; belly; ankles; spine; psoas
Level: Advanced
Sanskrit Name: *Padma Sarvangasana*
Time: 30 seconds to a minute in each stage
Indications: Stretching; strengthening; stimulation
Contraindications: High blood pressure; spine injuries; shoulder injuries

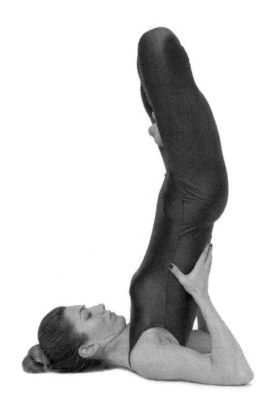

The Lotus Shoulderstand is an advanced inversion pose that stimulates the thyroid gland, kidneys, and belly organs; strengthens the back muscles; and stretches the ankles, spine, and psoas.

To perform this exercise, you must:

1. Lie prone, belly up, and perform the Supported Shoulderstand Pose.
2. While supporting your back with your hands, bring your legs into the Lotus Pose. Do this by slightly bending your knees, bringing your feet in front of your knees toward your pelvis.

153

3. Try to bend your knees as much as you can to hook your feet together just above the ankles, one on top of the other.
4. Hold this pose for 30 seconds to a minute. Breathe easily, and then turn your pelvis and legs towards the left. Support your left buttock with your left hand as you do.
5. Hold this pose for 30 seconds to a minute, and then repeat on the other side. Come up by unfolding your legs back into the Supported Shoulderstand Pose, and then come down as recommended in that pose.

Scorpion Pose

Focus: Back; elbows; spine
Level: Advanced
Sanskrit Name: *Vrishchikasana*
Time: 30 seconds, up to 3 minutes
Indications: Stretching; toning; stimulation
Contraindications: Spine injuries; shoulder injuries; elbow injuries; high blood pressure

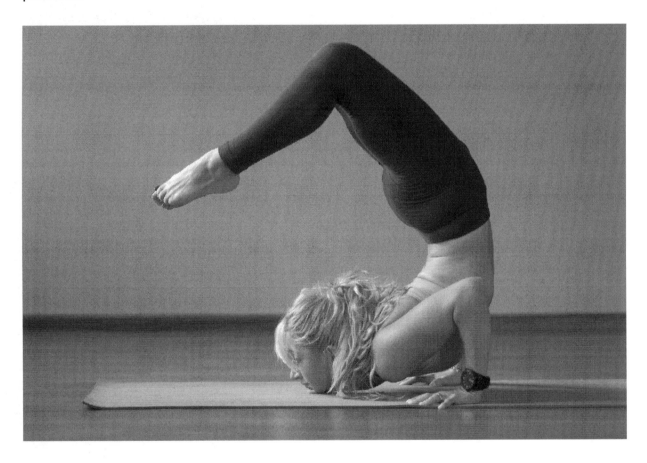

The Scorpion is an advanced inverted pose that increases the flow of fresh blood to the brain; stimulates the nerves; tones the back muscles; and stretches the spine.

To perform this exercise, you must:

1. Part from the Headstand Pose.
2. Relax your body, bend your knees, and arch your back. You will have to slowly shift your hands so that your weight rests on your forearms. To maintain your balance, do this with the utmost care and without rushing. Keep your hands parallel and close to each other to support your body.
3. Relax your body as much as you can, and try to arch your back even further. If you're flexible and strong enough, you can drop your legs further than your head. If not, you can keep your legs close and try to lift your head slightly to meet them.
4. Hold this pose for 30 seconds initially. You can gradually increase your stay up to 3 minutes. Come off the position by returning to the Headstand Pose, and then coming off it in the recommended manner.

Performing the Mountain Pose for 30 seconds after the Scorpion Pose helps balance the blood distribution again.

Headstand Pose

Focus: Abdomen; back
Level: Advanced
Sanskrit Name: *Shirshasana*
Time: 30 seconds to a minute, up to 3 minutes
Indications: Improves balance; stimulates; toning
Contraindications: High blood pressure; spine injuries; dizziness

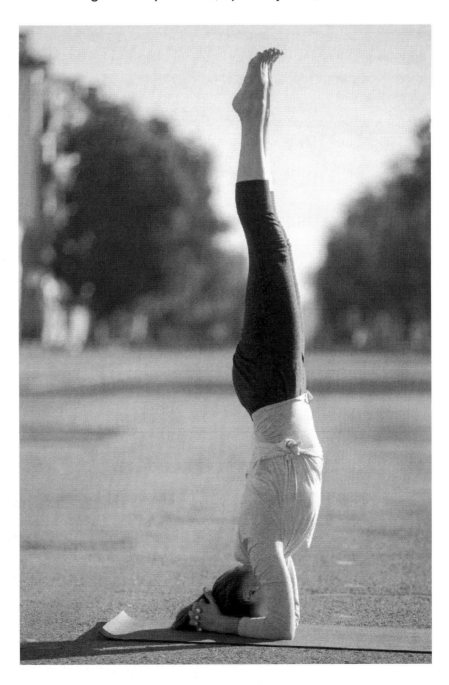

The Headstand Pose is a tough pose that shifts the body upside down and places the weight on the crown of the head.

It increases the blood supply to the head; improves balance, focus, and memory; stimulates the sensory organs; and tones the abdominal and back muscles.

To perform this exercise, you must:

1. Part from the Diamond Pose, resting your hands on your thighs.
2. Breathe easily and rest your head on the floor just in front of your knees. Clasp your fingers behind your head and support the back of your head with your palms. Keep your forearms resting on the floor, forming a triangle with your head.
3. Curl your toes under, lift your hips, and extend your legs. Focus on the balance of your body. Try walking your feet closer so that your buttocks are high above your head.
4. Shift your weight onto your forearms and lift your feet from the floor. Keeping your back as straight as you can, bring your heels towards your buttocks.
5. Extend your legs fully, keeping your feet relaxed and upright. Balance your body weight between your head, neck, and forearms.
6. Hold the pose for 30 seconds to a minute. Gradually increase your stay, up to 3 or so minutes, but don't go beyond 5 minutes. Come down by bending your knees, placing your feet down and then sitting on your buttocks again, returning to the Diamond Pose.

Yoga Poses for the Hips

Fire Log Pose

Focus: Hip; groins
Level: Beginner
Sanskrit Name: *Agnistambhasana*
Time: At least a minute
Indications: Stretching
Contraindications: Knee injuries; back injuries

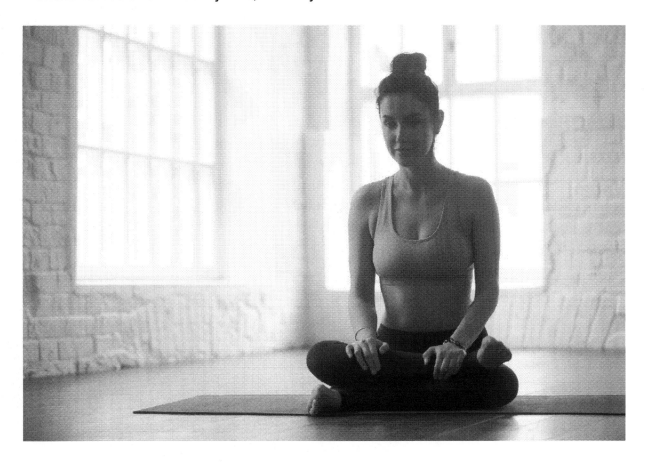

The Fire Log Pose is a seated pose that gives a thorough stretch to the outer hips and groins. It has been reported as therapeutic for sciatic pain.

To perform this exercise, you must:

1. Sit on the floor. You might want to roll out a couple of thickly-folded blankets beforehand to make the pose more comfortable for you.

2. Bend your knees and rest your soles flat on the floor.
3. Gently shrug your shoulders, and then firmly roll the heads of your upper arm bones back in. Press the bottom tips of your shoulder blades into your back.
4. Move your left foot under your right leg to the outside of your right hip, laying the outer leg on the floor as you do. Now, stack your right leg on top of the left, making sure that your right ankle is just outside your left knee (making the sole perpendicular to the floor).
5. If you're flexible enough in the hips, try sliding your left shin forward, just below the right. This will make the exercise more challenging. If you're not, keep your left heel beside your right hip.
6. Beginners are often tight in the hips. If this is your case, bringing the ankle to the outer knee will be too hard, so instead, sit with your shins crossed, just like in the Easy Pose.
7. Push your heels and spread your toes. Keeping your torso as long as you can, proceed to lean forward from your groins. Don't put too much compression on your belly, and keep the space between your pubis and navel long.
8. Lay your hands down on the ground in front of your shins.
9. As you inhale, your torso should raise slightly. Inhale and lengthen from your pubis to your sternum. Fold deeper on the next exhalation.
10. Hold the pose for at least a minute, more if you want. Come out by uncrossing your legs while keeping your torso upright. Repeat the exercise with your legs reversed for the same length of time.

Lotus Pose

Focus: Spine; pelvis; abdomen; knees; ankles
Level: Intermediate
Sanskrit Name: *Padmasana*
Time: 10 seconds to a minute
Indications: Stretching; stimulation; mental relaxation
Contraindications: Knee injuries; ankle injuries

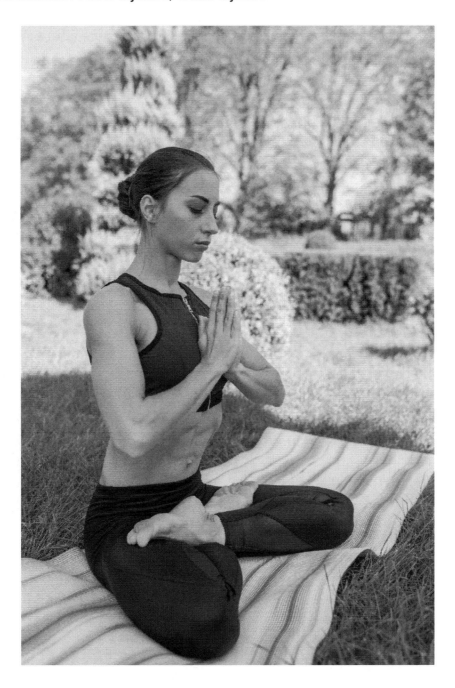

The Lotus Pose is an intermediate-advanced meditative pose that soothes the mind; stimulates the pelvis, spine, and abdomen; and stretches the knees and ankles.

To perform this exercise, you must:

1. Sit on the floor with your legs stretched in front of you. Bend your right knee, bringing the lower leg into a cradle. The outer edge of your foot should be notched into the crook of your left elbow while your knee is wedged into the crook of your right elbow.
2. Clasp your hands outside of your shin if possible. Lean your front torso toward your inner right leg so that you lengthen your spine.
3. Sway your leg back and forth to get a feel of the full movement range of your hip joint.
4. Bend your left knee to turn the leg out. Move your right leg far to the right, locking the knee tight by pressing the back of the thigh into the calf.
5. Swing your leg across in front of your torso, swiveling from the hip and not the knee. Nestle the outside edge of the foot into your inner left groin. Bring your right knee as close to the left as you can, pressing your right heel into your left lower belly as you do. Your sole should be *perpendicular*, not parallel, to the floor.
6. Lean back to lift your right leg off the floor, and then lift the left in front of the right. To achieve this, you must hold the underside of your left shin in your hands. Slide your left leg over the right carefully; you must snuggle the edge of your left foot into your right groin.
7. Swivel into position from the hip joint and press your heel evenly against your lower belly. Arrange the sole perpendicular to the floor.
8. Draw your knees as close together as you can, and then use the edges of your feet to press your groins into the floor, lifting your sternum as you do.
9. If you want, you can place your hands in the Jnana Mudra: palms facing toward the ceiling while you touch your thumbs with your first fingers.
10. In the beginning, don't hold the pose more than 10 or 15 seconds. The Lotus Pose demands a lot of practice. Don't forget that once you come up, you must perform the exercise with your legs reversed. Gradually increase your stay up to a minute or so.

Revolved Triangle Pose

Focus: Legs; hips; spine
Level: Beginner
Sanskrit Name: *Parivrtta Trikonasana*
Time: 30 seconds to a minute per side
Indications: Strengthening; stretching; improves balance; opens chest
Contraindications: Headache (or migraine); insomnia; low blood pressure; diarrhea

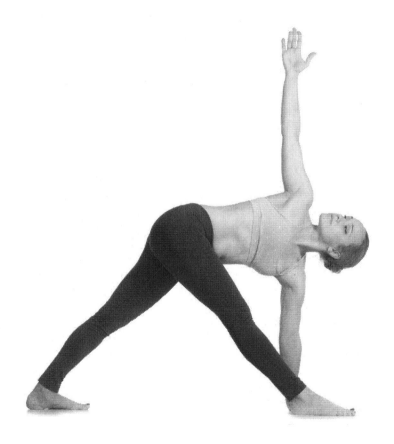

The Revolved Triangle Pose is a primordial pose for practice. Those who wish to execute the more complex poses will need to get familiar with this pose.

It stretches the hips and spine, strengthens the legs, opens the chest, and improves balance.

To perform this exercise, you must:

1. Start from the Mountain Pose. Exhale all the air from your lungs and then step your feet a little more than shoulder-width apart, about 3-and-a-half to 4 feet.

2. Lift your arms parallel to the floor and then reach out to the sides, shoulder blades wide.
3. Turn your left foot 45° or 60° to the right and your right foot to the right about 90°.
4. Align your heels.
5. Turn your torso to the right, squaring your hip points as much as possible. Keep your left heel firmly grounded.
6. Exhaling all the air you can, lean your torso forward over the front leg, reaching your left hand down to the floor (or a block if you can't reach it) and your right hand up to the ceiling.
7. Beginners will probably feel their right hip slipping out to the side, or their torso hunching over the front leg. To alleviate this, press the right thigh actively to the left and release the right hip from the right shoulder.
8. Starting out, gaze straight forward or to the floor. Looking up to your right hand might make you lose balance or even get dizzy.
9. You should stay between 30 seconds and one minute in this pose. Once ready, switch to the other side.

Practicing this pose regularly will help you perform the following poses with ease. Just 3 breaths should be enough. If you're feeling too uncomfortable, end prematurely.

Intense Side Stretch Pose

Focus: Spine; shoulders; legs; wrists; hips; hamstrings
Level: Intermediate
Sanskrit Name: *Parsvottanasana*
Time: 15 to 30 seconds
Indications: Stretching; strengthening; mental relaxation; abdominal stimulation; improves pose; improves balance; improves digestion
Contraindications: High blood pressure; back injuries

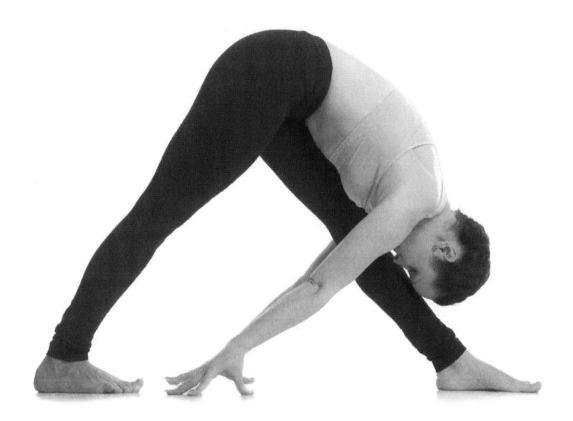

The Intense Side Stretch Pose is a deep side stretch pose that stretches the spine, shoulders, wrists, hips, and hamstrings. It's a great exercise to strengthen the legs, and to improve pose and balance.

To perform this exercise, you must:

1. Part from the Mountain Pose, stepping your feet about 3-and-a-half to 4 feet apart.

2. Place your hands on your hips and turn your left foot 45° to 60° to the right, while turning your right foot all the way out to the right (90°). Align your heels, firm your thighs, and center your right kneecap with your right ankle by turning your right thigh out.

3. Rotate your torso to the right, and as your left hip point turns, press the head of your left femur back into the ground, toward the back heel.

4. Push your outer thighs inward, as if you were wedging a block between your thighs. Firm your shoulder blades against your back and lengthen your coccyx toward the floor, arching the back of your upper torso slightly.

5. Lean your torso forward from your groins over your right leg until your torso is parallel to the ground. Push your fingertips into the floor on either side of your right foot. If you can't quite touch the floor with your hands, use a support, such as a pair of blocks, or the seat of a chair.

6. Push your thighs back, lengthening your torso forward through the top of the sternum with a lift.

7. During this pose, the front-leg hip tends to lift toward the shoulder, swinging out to the side, and shortening the front-leg side. Avoid this by softening the front-leg hip toward the ground, away from the same-side shoulder, while you continue to nestle the outer thighs.

8. Push the base of your big toe and the inner heel of your front foot firmly against the floor, lifting the inner groin of the front leg deep into your pelvis.

9. Hold your torso and head parallel to the ground for a few breaths, and if you're able, bring your torso even closer to the top of your thigh, without rounding from the waist. Eventually, your torso will rest down on the thigh.

10. Hold the pose for 15 to 30 seconds, and then come up by pressing actively through your back heel, dragging your coccyx down and into your pelvis.

Standing Forward Bend Pose

Focus: Hamstrings; calves; hips; knees; thighs
Level: Intermediate
Sanskrit Name: *Uttanasana*
Time: 30 seconds to a minute
Indications: Stretching; strengthening; abdominal stimulation; improves digestion
Contraindications: Back injury

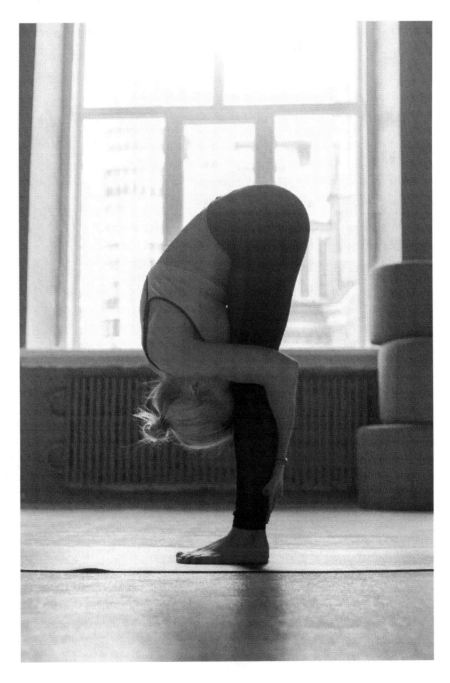

The Standing Forward Bend Pose is an exceptional restive pose that stretches the hamstrings, calves, and hips; strengthens the thighs and knees; stimulates the liver and kidneys; and relieves stress and mental fatigue.

Avoid this pose if you're in the process of healing back injuries.

To perform this exercise, you must:

1. Part from the Mountain Pose. Exhale all the air from your lungs and then bend forward, not from the waist but from the hip joints.
2. Draw your front torso out of your groins as you descend, opening the space between your pubis and top sternum. The goal here is lengthening your front torso as you move.
3. With your knees as straight as possible, bring your palms (or at least fingertips) to the front or the sides of your feet. If possible, bring your palms to the backs of your ankles. If not, crossing your forearms and holding your elbows will do.
4. Press your heels firmly against the floor and raise your sitting bones up.
5. Try lifting and lengthening your front torso slightly with each inhalation, doing the opposite with each exhalation.
6. To end, bring your hands back onto your hips and adjust the length of your front torso. Press your tailbone down into your pelvis and come up.

This pose is *typically* used to rest in between poses, but it can be practiced on its own. 30 seconds to 1 minute, 2 to 4 breaths, should be enough.

Extended Triangle Pose

Focus: Thighs; knees; ankles; groins; calves

Level: Intermediate

Sanskrit Name: *Utthita Trikonasana*

Time: 30 seconds to a minute per side

Indications: Stretching; strengthening; abdominal stimulation

Contraindications: Heart problems; diarrhea; headache; low (or high) blood pressure; neck injuries

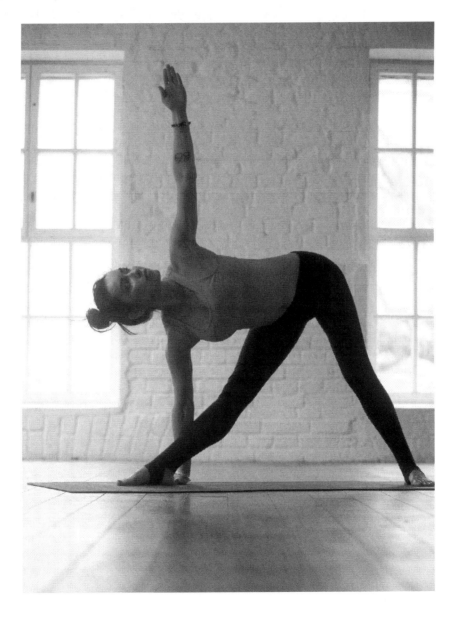

The Extended Triangle Pose is an essential intermediate pose that stretches and strengthens the thighs, knees, ankles, groins, and calves; stimulates the abdominal organs; relieves stress; and is therapeutic for flat feet, neck ache, and osteoporosis.

To perform this exercise, you must:

1. Part from the Mountain Pose, and separate your feet 3-and-a-half to 4 feet apart.
2. Lift your arms, making them parallel to the floor, and reach to the sides with your palms down, widening your shoulder blades.
3. Turn your left foot slightly to the right, and your right foot all the way to 90° right. Align both heels.
4. Firm your thighs and turn your right thigh outward, centering the kneecap with the ankle.
5. Extend your torso to the right, placing it directly over the plane of your right leg. Bend from the hip joint, not the waist.
6. Strengthen your left leg and press your outer heel firmly to the floor to anchor this movement.
7. Twist your torso to the left, but keep both sides equally long. The left hip should come slightly forward, to lengthen the tailbone toward the back heel.
8. Rest your right hand on your shin or ankle, or the floor outside your right foot. Try not to break the positioning of your torso.
9. Stretch your left arm up, toward the ceiling, keeping it centered with the tops of your shoulders.
10. Keep your head in a neutral position, or turn it to the left to gaze at your left thumb.
11. Hold the pose for 30 seconds to 1 minute. Come up by pressing the back heel into the floor, and then reaching the top arm up. Reverse feet and repeat for the same length of time.

Revolved Head to Knee Pose

Focus: Spine; hips; shoulders; hamstrings
Level: Advanced
Sanskrit Name: *Parivrtta Janu Sirsasana*
Time: One minute per side
Indications: Stretching; abdominal stimulation; improves digestion
Contraindications: Diarrhea; ankle injuries

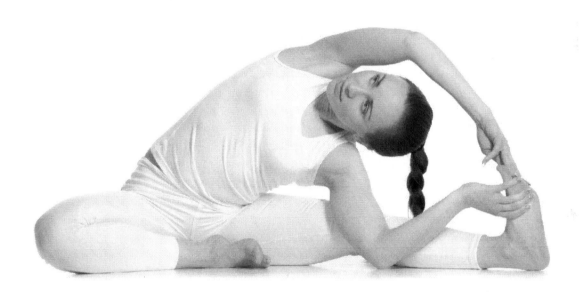

The Revolved Head to Knee Pose is the next level after the classic Head to Knee Forward Bend Pose. It stretches the spine, hips, shoulders, and hamstrings; stimulates the abdominal organs; and improves digestion.

1. Sit on the floor, with your torso upright and your legs wide, and bend your left knee, snuggling the heel with your left groin.
2. Slightly bend your right knee, and slide the heel a few inches toward your right buttock.
3. Lean to the right, pressing the back of your right shoulder against your inner right knee.

4. Lay your right forearm on the floor inside your right leg, palm facing up.
5. Lengthen the right side of your torso along the inside of your right thigh. Turn your right palm toward the inside edge of your right foot and take a hold of it, thumb down, on the top of the foot, with your fingers on the sole.
6. You must anchor this pose with the femur bone of your left leg. To do this, press your left femur firmly into the floor as you slowly extend your right knee. Keep the back of your shoulder connected to the inner knee as you extend.
7. Your torso will be dragged out by the straightening knee. When your knee is straightened, rotate your torso toward the ceiling.
8. Lift your left arm up toward the ceiling, leaning it back slightly, and then sweep it behind your left ear to take a grasp of your right foot.
9. Push your elbows away from each other to use them as a crank to increase the twist of your upper torso.
10. Turn your head up and look at the ceiling, or keep it in a neutral position.
11. Hold the pose for a minute. To come out, you must untwist your torso, but just before becoming upright, sweep it to the left, midway between your legs. Now you can lift it to an upright position. Repeat the exercise on the other side for the same time.

Horse Face Pose

Focus: Legs; knees; hips; thighs
Level: Intermediate
Sanskrit Name: *Vatayanasana*
Time: 30 seconds to a minute per side
Indications: Stretching; strengthening; abdominal stimulation
Contraindications: Knee injuries; ankle injuries; hip injuries

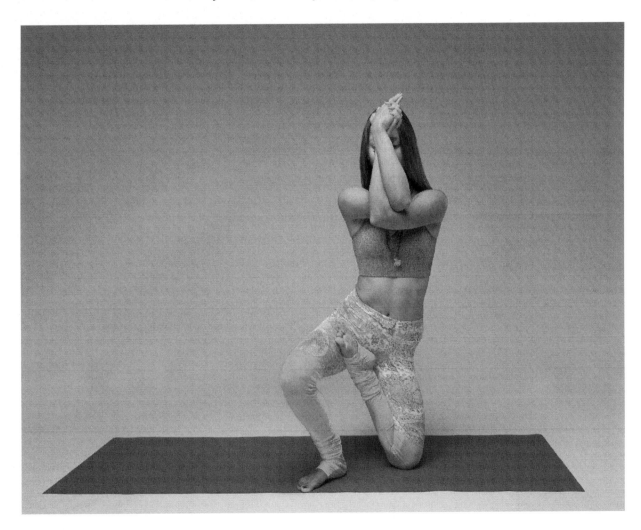

The Horse Face Pose is an intermediate pose that demands focus, strength, and will to perform.

It relieves tension from the sacroiliac region; stretches and strengthens the legs, knees, and hips; corrects the alignment between the hips and thighs; and helps reduce hyperactivity of the kidneys.

To perform this exercise, you must:

1. Stand upright, with your feet a little less than hip-width apart.
2. Deeply bend your left knee and prop your left foot against your inner right thigh. Hold your left ankle until you steady your body.
3. Focusing on your balance, slowly bend your right knee down, lowering your body to the floor. Rest the top of your left knee on the floor just near your right foot. Straighten your back and keep your torso balanced; don't tilt forward.
4. Bend your elbows; raise the left one to chest-level, and encircle your left hand with your right, joining the palms.
5. Hold this pose for 30 seconds to a minute, breathing easily. Unfold your arms, slowly come back up into the neutral standing position, and take a few breaths. Repeat the exercise with the arms and legs reversed for the same length of time.

Those with delicate knee joints should stay away from this pose.

Wide-Legged Forward Bend Pose

Focus: Legs; spine; hips
Level: Advanced
Sanskrit Name: *Prasarita Padottanasana*
Time: Up to a minute
Indications: Strengthening; abdominal stimulation
Contraindications: Back injuries

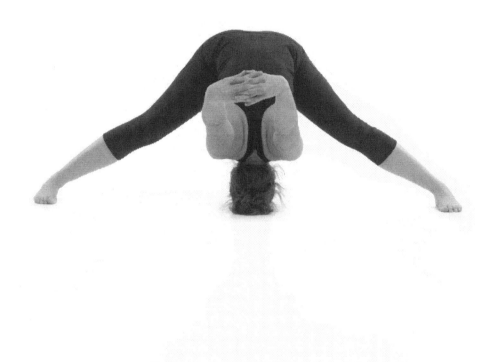

The Wide-Legged Forward Bend Pose is a much wider forward bend that builds up a lot of strength and endurance. It strengthens the hips, legs and spine, and stimulates the belly organs.

To perform this exercise, you must:

1. Part from the Mountain Pose, then put your feet 3 to 4-and-a-half feet apart. Place your hands on your hips while adjusting your inner feet so that they're parallel to each other.
2. Raise your inner arches by drawing up on your ankles, then press the outermost edges of your feet firmly into the floor. Engage your thigh muscles by drawing them up.
3. Lift your chest and lengthen your torso so that the front is slightly longer than the back.
4. Lean your torso forward from your hip joints while maintaining the length. As it becomes parallel, press your hands onto the floor below your shoulders and extend your elbows fully.
5. At this point, your legs and arms should be perpendicular to the floor. Move your spine evenly into your back torso so that your back is a bit concave from the tailbone to the skull.
6. Lift your head and direct your gaze toward the ceiling.
7. Press your top thighs back to lengthen your front torso. Drag your inner groins away from each other to widen the base of your pelvis. While keeping the concavity, walk your fingers between your feet, and then bend your elbows to form a full forward bend. Keep your front torso as long as possible while resting the crown of your head on the floor if possible.
8. Push your inner palms into the floor, fingers pointing forward. If you're flexible enough, you can try moving your hands back until your forearms are perpendicular to the floor with your upper arms parallel. If doing so, keep your arms parallel to each other, with your shoulder blades widened across your back and away from your ears.
9. Hold the pose for as long as a minute. End by bringing your hands back onto the floor below your shoulders to push and lengthen your front torso.

Eagle Pose

Focus: Ankles; calves; thighs; hips; shoulders
Level: Advanced
Sanskrit Name: *Garudasana*
Time: 15 to 30 seconds per side
Indications: Stretching; strengthening
Contraindications: Knee injuries

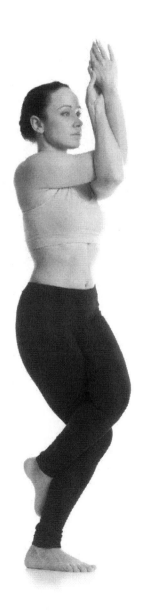

The Eagle Pose is a demanding pose that requires strength, flexibility, and lots of endurance and concentration. It strengthens and stretches the ankles, calves, thighs, hips, and shoulders.

To perform this exercise, you must:

1. Part from the Mountain Pose, and then bend your knees slightly, lifting your left foot up while you cross your left thigh over the right. The tricky part is doing all this while balancing on your right foot.
2. Point your left toes toward the floor, push your left foot back, and then hook the top of the foot behind the lowermost part of your right calf.
3. Extend your arms forward, parallel to the floor, and then widen your shoulder blades across the back of your torso. Cross your arms in front of your torso so that the right is above the left, and then bend your elbows.
4. Nestle your right elbow into the crook of the left and raise your forearms perpendicular to the floor. The backs of your hands should face each other.
5. Push your right hand to the right, and your left hand to the left, so that your palms face each other. The thumb of the right hand should cross in front of the pinky of the left one. Now press your palms against each other as much as you can. Raise your elbows and stretch your fingertips toward the ceiling.
6. Hold the pose for 15 to 30 seconds. End by unwinding your legs and arms and stepping back into the Mountain Pose, then repeat for the same time with legs and arms reversed.

Yoga Poses for the Legs

Upward Extended Feet Pose

Focus: Back; abdomen; psoas; legs
Level: Beginner
Sanskrit Name: *Urdhva Prasarita Padasana*
Time: 5 seconds to a minute in each stage
Indications: Strengthening; toning; improves pose
Contraindications: Back injuries; hip injuries

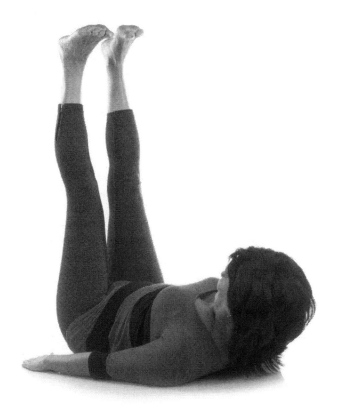

The Upward Extended Feet Pose is a leg stretching pose that strengthens the core muscles; stretches the ankles, thighs, spine, and calves; tones and reduces the fat in the belly; and improves the flexibility of the psoas.

To perform this exercise, you must:

1. Lie prone on the floor, belly up. Keep your arms beside you, either alongside your ears, or down along the sides of your torso.
2. Firm the core muscles of your abs and push your navel down toward your spine. Push the sides of your waist into the floor.
3. Exhale slowly as you raise both your legs off the ground. Be sure to keep your spine straight and pressed down into the floor.
4. Swing your legs up toward the ceiling, keeping them perpendicular relative to the floor. Stretch through your inner thighs, up to your toes. Hold this pose for 5 to 10 seconds.
5. Angle your legs about a third down, and hold the pose for 5 to 10 seconds. It's okay if your lower back raises slightly from the floor.
6. Angle your legs down even a little more, keeping them a few inches off the ground. Hold the pose for 5 to 10 seconds.
7. If you have some abdominal endurance remaining, you can swing your legs back up to perpendicular. If you feel spent, lower your legs to the floor and rest a little before repeating the exercise.
8. Gradually increase your stay in each stage until you can hold each one for about a minute.

Dolphin Pose

Focus: Shoulders; hamstrings; calves; arches; legs; arms
Level: Intermediate
Sanskrit Name: *Ardha Pincha Mayurasana*
Time: 30 seconds to a minute
Indications: Stretching; strengthening; improves digestion; mental relaxation
Contraindications: Neck injuries; shoulder injuries

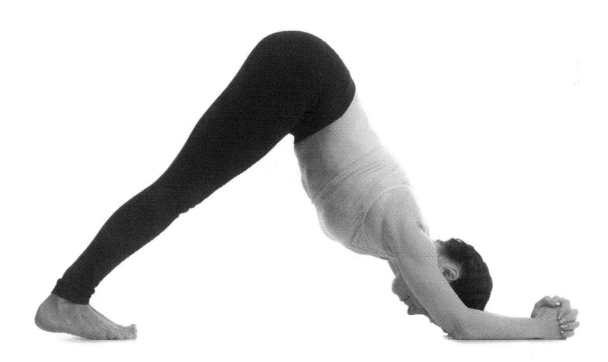

The Dolphin Pose is a nice shoulder-opening pose that strengthens the arms, legs, hamstrings, calves, and arches. It is regarded as therapeutic for conditions such as headache, insomnia, and back pain.

To perform this exercise, you must:

1. Get down to the floor on your hands and knees.
2. Place your knees directly below your hips, with your forearms on the floor and your shoulders above your wrists. Secure your forearms into the floor by firmly clasping your hands together.

3. Curl your toes under and lift your knees off the ground with an exhale. Initially, your knees should be *slightly* bent, and your heels should be off the floor.
4. Lengthen your tailbone away from the back of your pelvis, and then press it lightly toward your pubis. Lift your sitting bones toward the ceiling, and then drag your inner legs up into your groins through your inner ankles. Actively press your forearms into the floor.
5. Firm your shoulder blades into your back, and then broaden them away from your spine, drawing them toward your tailbone.
6. Set your head between your upper arms. Don't let it hang or press into the floor.
7. Try straightening your knees as much as you can, making sure that your upper back doesn't round. If it rounds, keep your legs bent.
8. Keep lengthening your tailbone away from your pelvis, and then lift the top of your sternum away from the floor.
9. Hold the pose for 30 seconds to a minute. End by exhaling and calmly releasing your knees to the floor.

Side Reclining Leg Lift Pose

Focus: Legs; torso sides; belly
Level: Intermediate
Sanskrit Name: *Anantasana*
Time: 30 seconds to a minute
Indications: Stretching; toning
Contraindications: Spine injuries

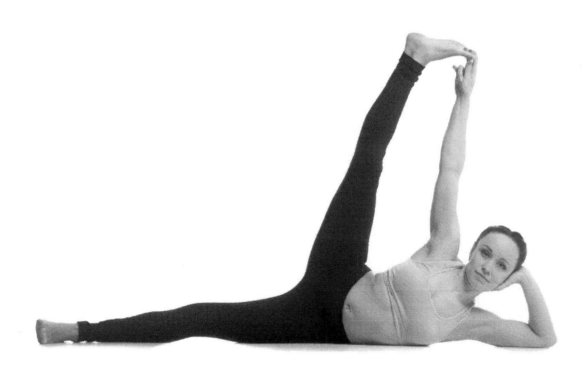

The Side Reclining Leg Lift Pose is an intermediate reclining pose to stretch the lower side of the body, especially the backs of the legs, as well as to tone the abdomen.
To perform this exercise, you must:

1. Lie on the floor on top of your right side. Press through your right heel, flexing the ankle, and use the outer edge of the foot to stabilize your position. If you still feel a bit unstable, prop your soles against a nearby wall.

2. Extend your right arm out along the floor, parallel to your torso, making a long line from your heels to your fingertips.
3. Bend your right elbow and hold your head in your palm. Slide the elbow away from your torso and stretch the armpit.
4. Rotate your left leg so that the toes point toward the ceiling. Bend and draw the knee toward your torso, reaching across the inside of the leg to take a hold of your left big toe with your index and middle fingers. Stabilize your grip by wrapping your thumb around your fingers. If this is not possible for you, loop a strap around the sole and hold it firmly.
5. Inhale, and then extend your leg up toward the ceiling.
6. The lifted leg will angle a bit forward most of the time, and your top buttock might drop back. To avoid this, firm your sacrum against your pelvis. This will allow you to move your leg slightly back toward a perpendicular placement relative to the floor. Push actively through both heels.
7. Hold the pose for 30 seconds to a minute. End by releasing the leg, taking a few breaths, and then rolling over onto your left side. Repeat the exercise on the other side for the same length of time.

Reclining Hand to Toe Pose

Focus: Calves; groins; hamstrings; hips; thighs
Level: Beginner
Sanskrit Name: *Supta Padangusthasana*
Time: At least a minute, up to 3 in the final stage
Indications: Strengthening; stretching; improves digestion
Contraindications: Diarrhea; high blood pressure; headache

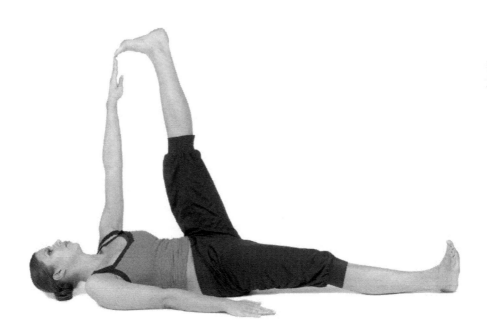

The Reclining Hand to Toe Pose is a cool restorative pose that will help you deal with debilitating backaches and tight hamstrings.

It stretches the hips, thighs, hamstrings, groins, and calves with the help of a strap or a belt.

To perform this exercise, you must:

1. Lie prone on the ground, face up. You might want to roll out a folded blanket or something like that to keep your head resting comfortably.

2. Stretch your legs thoroughly and then bend your left knee toward you, drawing the thigh into your torso.
3. Once your left thigh is hugging your belly, press your right thigh into the floor and loop a strap around the arch of your left foot. Hold it with both hands, inhale, and then straighten the knee, pressing your heel toward the ceiling. Keep recoiling the strap until your elbows are completely stretched.
4. Broaden your shoulder blades across your back and keep your hands as high on the strap as you can. Then press your shoulder blades into the floor, widening your collarbones away from your sternum.
5. Once your leg is extended perpendicular to the floor, start drawing your foot closer to your head to stretch the back of the leg.
6. At this point, feel free to stay in this position. You can also turn the leg outwards so that your knee and toes look left. After some time, sway your leg to the left, holding it just inches above the floor. Feel free to rotate as much as you want to relieve tension.
7. To get your leg back to vertical, lighten the grip of the straps and let your leg carry itself back up.
8. Now hold the pose. Once ready, rest your leg in place for 30 seconds, and then repeat on the other leg for the same time.

The goal here is twofold: first, to increase your flexibility to the point you can grip your toes without a strap; second, to gradually increase the duration you can spend in this exercise.

You should spend at least a minute in the final stage, eventually reaching 3 minutes max. Taking even breaths will help you endure the pressure.

Reclining Bound Angle Pose

Focus: Inner thighs; groins; knees
Level: Intermediate
Sanskrit Name: *Supta Baddha Konasana*
Time: 1 minute, up to 10
Indications: Stretching; abdominal stimulation
Contraindications: Groin injury; knee injury

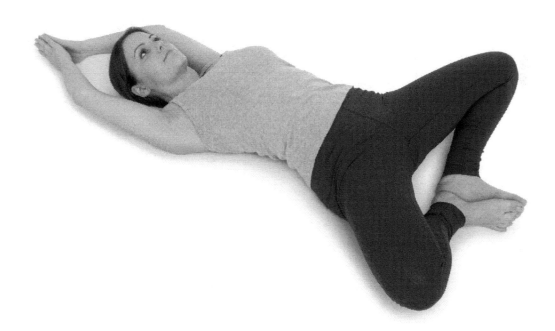

The Reclining Bound Angle Pose is a restorative pose that stimulates the abdominal organs and heart; stretches the inner thighs, groins, and knees; and relieves stress and fatigue.

To perform this exercise, you must:

1. Part from the Bound Angle Pose. Lean your torso back toward the ground, leaning first on your hands, then on your forearms. Spread your pelvis and release your lower back and upper buttocks through your tailbone.

187

2. Rest your torso all the way to the floor. Rolling up a folded blanket to rest your head and neck on might be a good idea.
3. Grip your thigh tops and rotate the insides externally, pressing the outer thighs from the hips to the knees, widening your knees away from your hips.
4. Slide your hands down along your inner thighs up to the groins.
5. Push your hip points together, widening the back pelvis as you narrow your front.
6. Place your arms on the floor so that they form a 45° angle with the sides of your torso. Keep your palms up.
7. Resist the urge to push your knees down. This will only harden your groins, belly, and lower back. You must consciously take control of your groins to drag them down into your pelvis.
8. Starting out, you might stay a minute, but you should gradually extend your stay up to 10 minutes. End by pressing your thighs together, then rolling onto one side, and finally pushing yourself away from the floor.

Half Moon Pose

Focus: Groins; hamstrings; calves; chest; ankles; thighs; spine
Level: Intermediate
Sanskrit Name: *Ardha Chandrasana*
Time: 30 seconds to a minute per side
Indications: Stretching; strengthening; improves digestion; improves balance
Contraindications: Headache (or migraine); diarrhea; insomnia; low blood pressure

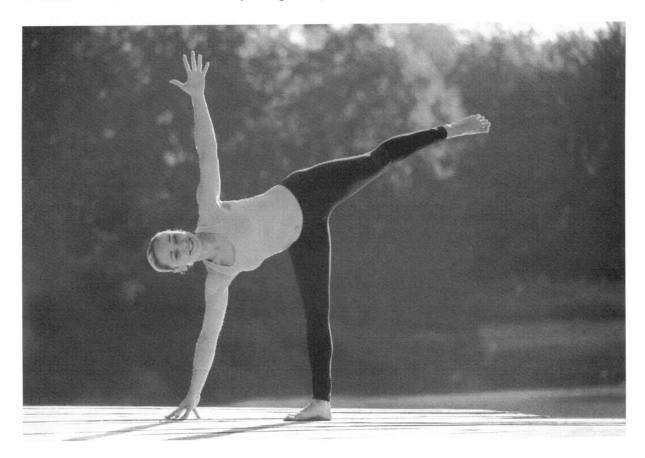

The Half Moon Pose is a symbolic balancing pose that stretches the groins, hamstrings, calves, and chest; strengthens the abdomen, ankles, thighs, and spine; and improves coordination, stability, and balance.

1. Part from the Extended Triangle Pose, leaning to the right side, with your left hand resting on your left hip.
2. Bend your right knee and slide your left foot about 6 to 12 inches forward along the ground. As you do it, reach your right hand forward, at least 12 inches beyond the outer edge of your right foot (little-toe side).

3. Press your right hand and heel firmly into the ground and straighten your right leg while you lift your left leg parallel (or slightly above it) to the floor.
4. Stretch through your left heel actively to firm the raised leg. Do so without locking the standing knee; make sure it remains aligned forward without being turned inward.
5. Twist your upper torso to the left, but keep your left hip moving forward. Keep your left hand on your left hip, and place yourself in a neutral position, looking forward.
6. Bear your weight on the standing leg. Press the lower hand gently into the floor, using it to regulate your balance.
7. Lift the inner ankle of the standing foot up, as if pulling energy from the ground into your groin.
8. Nestle your sacrum and shoulder blades firmly against your back torso and lengthen your coccyx toward the raised heel.
9. Hold the pose for 30 seconds to a minute. Take a few breaths as you lower the raised leg to the floor, and then return to the Extended Triangle Pose. Perform the exercise once again, with the feet reversed, for the same length of time.

Extended Hand to Toe Pose

Focus: Legs; ankles; arms; back
Level: Intermediate
Sanskrit Name: *Utthita Hasta Padangustasana*
Time: 15 to 30 seconds per side
Indications: Stretching; strengthening; improves balance
Contraindications: Ankle injuries; back injuries

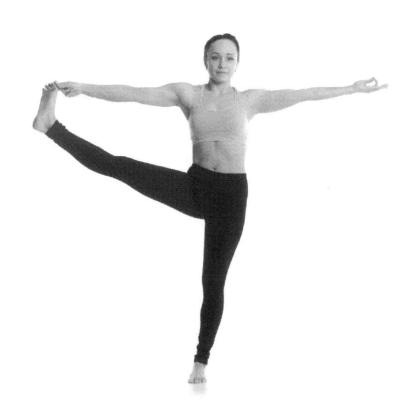

The Extended Hand to Toe Pose is an intermediate side stretch that demands a great deal of balance and concentration.

It stretches the backs of the legs, improves your balance, and strengthens your ankles and legs.

To perform this exercise, you must:

1. Part from the Mountain Pose and bend your right knee, bringing it toward your belly.
2. Reach your left arm alongside your thigh, cross it over the front ankle, and grasp the outside of your left foot. If you can't comfortably hold your foot, loop a strap around the sole and hang onto it.
3. Firm the front thigh of the standing leg, and push the outer thigh inward.
4. Inhale deeply and stretch your left leg forward. Straighten your knee as much as you can. If your position is steady enough, swing the raised leg out to the side. Consciously control your breathing, as this helps you secure your balance.
5. Hold the pose for 15 to 30 seconds. Inhale, lower the raised leg, and repeat the exercise with the other leg for the same length of time.

Reclining Hero Pose

Focus: Abdomen; thighs; psoas; knees; ankles; arches; legs
Level: Intermediate
Sanskrit Name: *Supta Virasana*
Time: At least 30 seconds, up to 5 minutes
Indications: Stretching; strengthening; improves digestion
Contraindications: Back injuries; knee injuries; ankle injuries

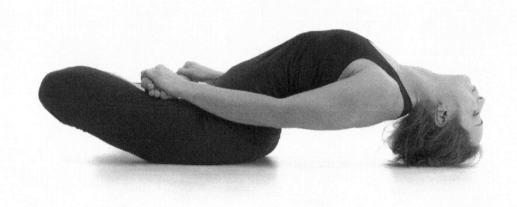

The Reclining Hero Pose is a reclined version of the Hero Pose. It steps back to bring the thigh and ankle stretch to the next level.

To perform this exercise, you must:

1. Part from the Hero Pose, and then lower your back torso toward the floor.
2. Lean onto your hands, then your forearms and elbows.
3. Once you're leaning on your elbows, place your hands on the back of your pelvis, and then release your lower back and buttocks by spreading them down toward the tailbone. Now finish reclining. Beginners might prefer using a support like stacked folded blankets or a bolster instead of the ground.
4. If your groins are tight, your front pelvis will be dragged toward your knees, and your belly and lower back will tense in consequence. Use your hands to pull your front ribs down, and then lift your pubis toward your navel. If that isn't enough to lengthen your lower back toward the floor, it would be best to use a higher support.
5. Lay your arms and hands on the floor, angled at 45° from the sides of your torso, palms up.
6. Push the heads of your thigh bones deep into your hip sockets. If you need to, you can lift your knees slightly to soften your groins. You can also allow some free space between your knees, as long as you can keep your thighs parallel to each other. Be sure that the distance between your knees isn't greater than hip-width.
7. Hold the pose for 30 seconds to a minute while you're starting out, but gradually increase your stay (by 5 or 10 seconds) up to 5 minutes. End by pressing your forearms into the floor, and then coming up onto your hands.

Wide-Angle Seated Forward Bend Pose

Focus: Legs; spine; groins
Level: Intermediate
Sanskrit Name: *Upavistha Konasana*
Time: 10 seconds to a minute
Indications: Stretching; strengthening; abdominal stimulation
Contraindications: Back injury

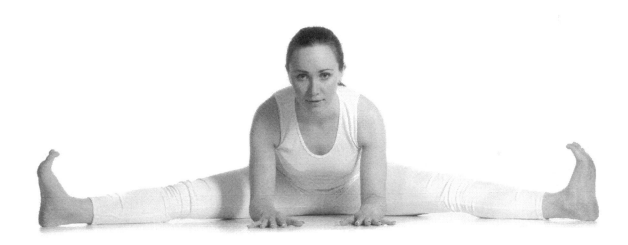

The Wide-Angle Seated Forward Bend Pose is a tougher forward bend that stretches the legs thoroughly, strengthens the spine, stimulates the abdominal organs, and relieves mental fatigue.

To perform this exercise, you must:

1. Part from the Staff Pose. Lean your torso back slightly on your hands.
2. Lift and open your legs into a 90° angle.

3. Push your hands into the floor and then slide your buttocks forward to widen your legs another 10° or 20°. If your buttocks aren't resting comfortably on the floor, slide a folded blanket underneath.

4. Turn your thighs outward and pin your outer thighs into the floor, pointing your kneecaps toward the ceiling. Stretch your soles through your heels.

5. Walk your hands forward between your legs, keeping your arms long as you do. Emphasize moving from the hip joints rather than the waist, and keep lengthening your front torso. If you start bending from the waist, stop and start lengthening from your pubis to your navel, continuing forward as far as possible.

6. Ideally, increase the bend after each exhalation until you feel comfortably stretched in the back of your legs. Hold the pose for a minute or longer.

Hand Under Foot Pose

Focus: Belly; thighs; ankles; arms; calves
Level: Intermediate
Sanskrit Name: *Padahastasana*
Time: 20 to 40 seconds
Indications: Stretching; strengthening; toning; abdominal stimulation
Contraindications: Heart problems; high blood pressure; spine injuries

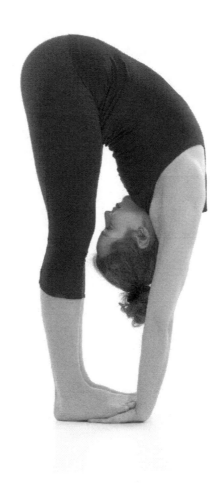

The Hand Under Foot Pose is an intermediate-advanced forward bend pose that tones the belly; stimulates the digestive organs; stretches the thighs, ankles, and arms; and strengthens the thigh and calf muscles.

To perform this exercise, you must:

1. Stand straight, with your torso upright. Your legs should be together, and your hands alongside your thighs.
2. Puff your chest, without tightening your body, and raise your hands straight up toward the ceiling. Make sure your biceps meet your ears. Keep your elbows extended and your palms forward.
3. Exhale, and bend forward from the lower back. Keep your legs straight and your knees unbent. Lower your whole back and hands on a single line until your upper body makes a 90° angle with your legs.
4. Keep lowering until your abdomen touches your thighs, followed by your chest.
5. Grasp each heel with the respective hand and try to touch your knees with your forehead.
6. Slide your fingers under your toes from the sides. Hold this pose for 5 to 15 seconds and then bend downward until you can reach your toes with your hands.
7. Hold this pose for 20 to 40 seconds.

Standing Split Pose

Focus: Hamstrings; calves; thighs; ankles; quads
Level: Advanced
Sanskrit Name: *Urdhva Prasarita Eka Padasana*
Time: 30 seconds to a minute per side
Indications: Stretching; strengthening; abdominal stimulation
Contraindications: Back injuries; ankle injuries; knee injuries

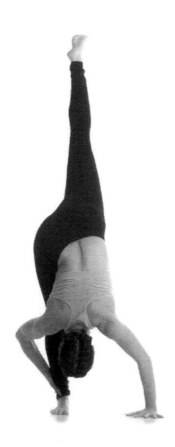

The Standing Split Pose is an advanced vertical split pose that focuses on the stretch of your quads and hamstrings. It strengthens the hamstrings, calves, thighs, and ankles and stimulates the abdominal organs.

To perform this exercise, you must:

1. Part from the Warrior II Pose, with your right leg forward.
2. Inhale deeply, and then cartwheel your left arm up and over your head, making an opening in your left ribs.

3. Exhale and turn your torso to the right, using the ball of your left foot as a pivot to lift your heel off the floor. Lean forward and try to nestle your front torso onto your right thigh, placing your hands on the floor at either side of your right foot. If your hands can't comfortably reach the ground, use a support such as two blocks, or two stacks of books.
4. Now comes a tricky part. You must walk your hands slightly ahead of your right foot to shift your weight onto the right leg. As you do, you must slowly straighten the leg, while lifting your left leg parallel to the floor.
5. Your left hip and leg might rotate slightly outward; this leads to lifting your hip away from the floor and angling your pelvis to the right. Avoid this by internally rotating your left thigh, keeping the front of your pelvis parallel to the floor.
6. The knee angle of the standing leg is important. Your knee might rotate inward, so be sure to rotate the thigh outward so that the kneecap faces straight forward.
7. The focus *is not* on how high your raised leg goes, but on how you direct energy into both legs. Your raised leg should be more or less parallel with your torso, meaning that it ascends as your torso descends. If you're flexible enough, you should be capable of reaching the back ankle of the standing leg with one of your hands.
8. Hold the pose for 30 seconds to a minute. End by slowly lowering the raised leg with an exhale, and then repeat the exercise on the other side for the same time.

Heron Pose

Focus: Hamstrings; abdomen
Level: Advanced
Sanskrit Name: *Krounchasana*
Time: 30 seconds to a minute per side
Indications: Stretching; abdominal stimulation
Contraindications: Knee injuries; ankle injuries; pregnancy

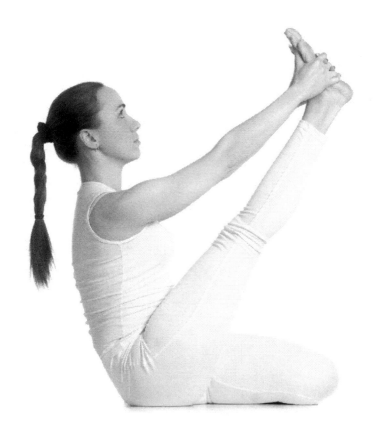

The Heron Pose is a challenging hamstring stretch that will demand superior thigh and groin strength.

1. Part from the Staff Pose, and then bring your left leg into the Reclining Hero Pose.
2. Bend your right knee and place your foot on the floor so that it sits just in front of your right sitting bone.
3. Rest your right arm against the inside of your right leg.
4. Cross your hand in front of your right ankle and grasp outside your right foot.
5. Reach and grasp your right foot with your left hand.

6. Lean back, but not too much so as to keep your front torso long. Firm your shoulder blades against your back to keep your chest lifted.
7. Raise your leg diagonally, forming a 45° angle relative to the floor. You can keep your leg lower than that, but try to keep your foot higher than or at least as high as your head level.
8. Hold the pose for 30 seconds to a minute. Then release the raised leg, carefully straightening the left leg. Take a few breaths, and then repeat the exercise on the other side for the same time.

Monkey Pose

Focus: Groins; hamstrings; thighs
Level: Advanced
Sanskrit Name: *Hanumanasana*
Time: 30 to a minute per side
Indications: Stretching; abdominal stimulation
Contraindications: Groin injuries; hamstring injuries

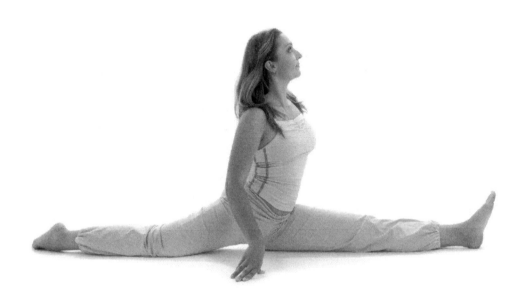

The Monkey Pose is an advanced pose that demands a lot of groin, hamstring, and thigh strength; it stretches these parts thoroughly and stimulates the abdominal organs.

Newcomers to the pose will have a hard time bringing their legs and pelvis down onto the floor. This stems from the tightness of the back of the legs and/or the front groins. Using a thick bolster or block below the pelvis, with the long axis parallel to your inner legs, will help you release your pelvis down during the exercise.

To perform this exercise, you must:

1. Kneel on the floor, then step your right foot forward about a foot or so in front of your left knee, and then rotate your right thigh out. Lift the inner sole away from the floor and then rest the foot on the outer edge of the heel.
2. Bend your torso forward, pressing your fingers into the floor. Slide your left knee back, straightening it as you descend your right thigh to the ground. Stop straightening the back knee before hitting the limit of your stretch.
3. Push your right heel away from your torso, gradually turning the front leg inward as it straightens to lift the kneecap toward the ceiling. As it straightens, continue pressing your left knee back, descending the front of your left thigh and the back of your right leg carefully into the floor. Be sure to center the right knee points directly up toward the ceiling.
4. Make sure that the back of the leg isn't angled out to the side; it should extend straight out of the hip. The center of the back kneecap should be sinking directly onto the floor. To keep the front leg active, extend through your heel, lifting your foot toward the ceiling. And then:
   a. Bring your hands into the *Anjali Mudra*: Clasp your palms together and rest your thumbs against your sternum.
   b. Extend your arms up toward the ceiling.
5. Hold the pose for 30 seconds to a whole minute. Come up by pressing your hands into the floor, lifting just enough to turn the front leg out slightly, and then return the front heel and the back knee to their starting positions. Reverse the legs and repeat for the same amount of time.

Yoga Poses for the Whole Body

Gate Pose

Focus: Torso; spine; hamstrings; shoulders
Level: Beginner
Sanskrit Name: *Parighasana*
Time: 30 seconds to a minute per side
Indications: Stretching; abdominal stimulation; opens shoulders
Contraindications: Knee injuries

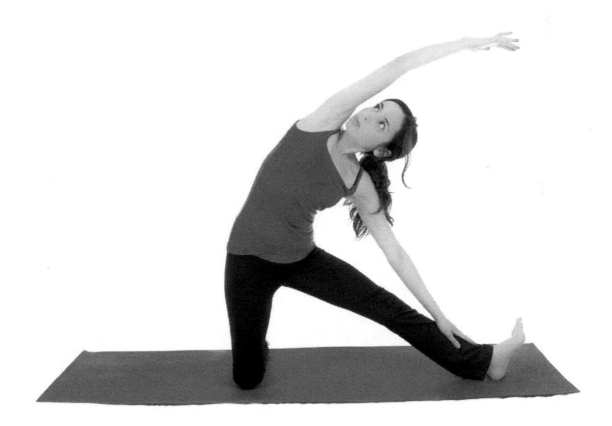

The Gate Pose is an excellent side body pose that stretches the sides of the torso, spine, and hamstrings; opens the shoulders; and stimulates the abdominal organs.

To perform this exercise, you must:

1. Kneel on the floor, extend your right leg out to the right, and press the foot against the ground.
2. Keep your left knee just below your left hip, so that its thigh remains perpendicular to the floor, and then align your heels.
3. Turn your pelvis slightly to the right, forcing your left hip point to come forward from the right, and turn your upper torso back to the left. Turn your right leg out so that your kneecap points at the ceiling.
4. Bring your arms out to your sides, keeping them parallel to the floor with the palms down.
5. Bend to the right, over the plane of your right leg, and lay your right hand down on your shin, your ankle, or the floor beside your outer right leg.
6. Compress the right side of your torso and stretch the left, resting your left hand on your outer left hip as you pull your pelvis down toward the ground.
7. Slip your hand up your lower left ribs, and then lift them toward your shoulder, making some space in your left waist.
8. Sweep your left arm over the back of your left ear. Most of the time, the side bend drops the torso down, so keeping your left hip in place, turn the upper torso away from the floor.
9. Hold the pose between 30 seconds and a minute. End by reaching through the top arm to draw your torso upright. Try to bring your right knee back beside the left, and repeat the exercise with your legs reversed.

This variation is more beginner-friendly. To perform the full side bend, you must part from step 4, and:

1. Tilt to the side over the straight leg.
2. Lower the underside of your torso as close as you can to the top of the straight leg.
3. Push the back of the lower hand onto the top of your foot, and sweet the top arm over your back, joining your palms.

If you have knee injuries, it's best to avoid this pose altogether. You can opt to perform the pose while sitting on a chair; you'll just have to arrange your legs in front of your torso, with your knees at right angles.

Bow Pose

Focus: Whole front body; ankles; thighs; groins; abdomen; psoas; chest
Level: Intermediate
Sanskrit Name: *Dhanurasana*
Time: 20 to 30 seconds, 2 to 3 times
Indications: Stretching; strengthening; abdominal stimulation; improves balance
Contraindications: Low (or high) blood pressure; migraine; insomnia; back injuries; neck injuries

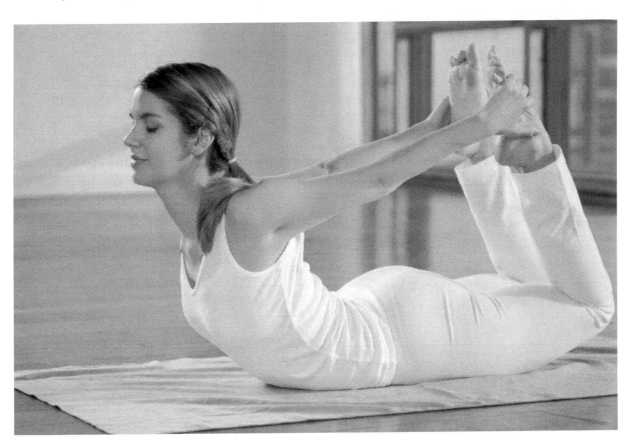

The Bow Pose is a deep backbend pose that stretches almost the entire body, including the ankles, groins, abdomen, chest, psoas, back muscles, and neck.

I suggest laying out a folded blanket to pad your torso and legs.

To perform this exercise, you must:

1. Lie on the floor with your belly down. Set your hands beside your torso, palms up.
2. Bend your knees, bringing your heels as close as possible to your buttocks. Reach back with your hands until you can take a hold of your ankles (not arches). Your knees shouldn't be wider than your hips. Try to keep them as hip-width as you can.
3. While clasping your ankles, lift your heels away from your buttocks while you lift your thighs from the floor to pull your upper torso and head off the ground. Sink your tailbone toward the floor and keep your back muscles soft. Press your shoulder blades into your back to open your heart as you lift your heels and thighs. Adjust your shoulder tops so that they're away from your ears, and look forward.
4. Don't stop breathing. You might be tempted to do so because the pressure between your belly and the floor makes it difficult, but you must try to breathe into the back of your torso.
5. Hold the pose between 20 and 30 seconds. End up by coming down and lying quietly. Take a few breaths and then repeat the pose once or twice more.

If holding your ankles is not possible, loop a strap around the front of them and hold the other end. Keep your arms extended and always try to walk closer and closer to your ankles with every practice.

King Pigeon Pose

Focus: Ankles; thighs; groins; abdomen; chest; neck; psoas; back
Level: Advanced
Sanskrit Name: *Kapotasana*
Time: At least 30 seconds
Indications: Stretching; strengthening; abdominal stimulation
Contraindications: Low (or high) blood pressure; migraine; insomnia; back injuries; neck injuries

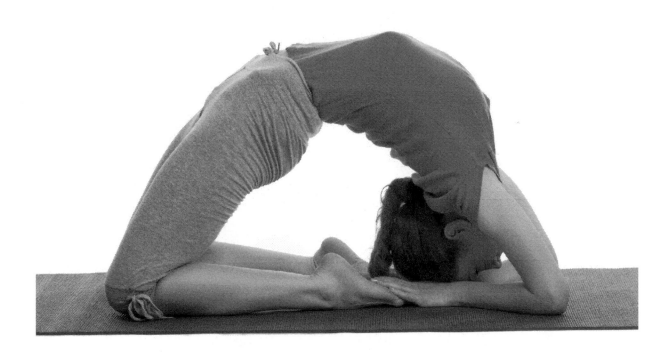

The King Pigeon Pose is an advanced pose that requires the endurance and flexibility of an advanced practitioner.

This pose stretches the entire front of the body, extending to the ankles, thighs, groins, abs, chest, and neck; unbends the psoas; strengthens the back muscles; and stimulates abdominal organs.

To perform this exercise, you must:

1. Kneel down, with your torso upright and your knees a bit narrower than hip-width apart. Keep your hips, shoulders, and head stacked directly above your knees.
2. Push the back of your pelvis down with your hands.
3. Slip your chin toward your sternum, and then lean your head and shoulders back as far as possible without moving your hips.
4. Firm your shoulder blades against your back and lift the top of your sternum. Once you've lifted your chest as much as you can, release your head back.
5. Before arching all the way back to place your head and hands on the ground, clasp your palms together in front of your sternum and perform the *Anjali Mudra* for a couple of breaths. Then separate your hands and reach them overhead toward the ground behind you. Bring your hips forward enough to counterbalance the backward movement of your torso and head, and keep your thighs as perpendicular as you can.
6. Bring your palms onto the floor and point your fingers toward your feet. Gently lower the crown of your head to the floor as well.
7. Expand your chest, taking a full inhalation, and then press your shins and forearms against the floor with a soft but thorough exhalation. Lengthen your tailbone toward your knees and lift your top sternum in the opposite direction.
8. Hold the pose for 30 seconds or more, expanding your chest a little more with each inhale as you soften your belly with each exhale. End by releasing your grip, walking your hands away from your feet, and then finally pushing your torso back to upright. Rest in the Child Pose for a few breaths.

Upward Facing Intense Pose

Focus: Whole backside; psoas; abdomen; spine; hamstrings
Level: Advanced
Sanskrit Name: *Urdhva Mukha Paschimottanasana*
Time: 30 seconds to a minute, up to 2 minutes
Indications: Stretching; strengthening; toning; abdominal stimulation
Contraindications: Knee injuries; back injuries; hamstring injuries

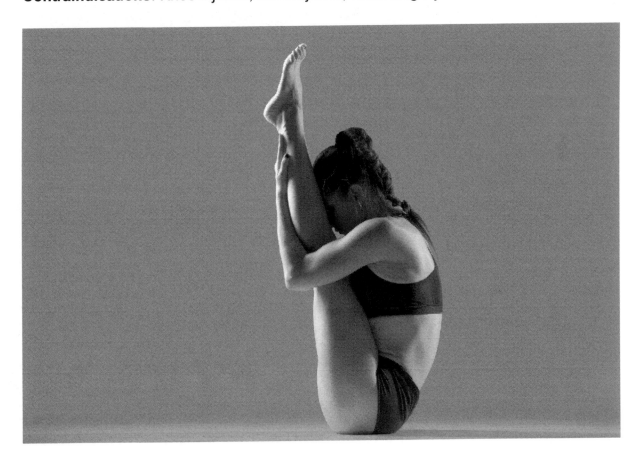

The Upward Facing Intense Pose is an advanced pose that stretches the entire backside.

It extends and strengthens the psoas, abdominals, hamstrings, and spine; alleviates backache; tones the belly; stimulates the digestive organs; and relieves tension from the back muscles.

To perform this exercise, you must:

1. Part from the Staff Pose, and then lie down on the ground. If you don't feel comfortable, slide a folded blanket or two underneath.
2. Inhale deeply and then lift your arms overhead. Exhale and then strongly raise your legs straight off the floor, reaching through your ankles.
3. Lift your hips and reach your hands toward your feet, clasping your big toes or soles with your fingers and securing the grip with your thumbs.
4. Inhale and curl in; you must focus on maintaining the balance of your body. Ideally, you should set your gaze upward, but if your neck is not comfortable, gazing forward is alright.
5. Exhale and try to meet your torso with your legs. Use the pressure from your limbs to maintain this position with balance. Try not to bend your knees while maintaining your back as straight as you can.
6. Hold the pose for 30 seconds to a minute. Gradually increase your stay to up to 2 minutes. Come down by gently releasing the grip from your toes, and then slowly releasing your legs onto the floor as you lower your torso.

Upward Facing Two Foot Staff Pose

Focus: Whole front body
Level: Advanced
Sanskrit Name: *Dwi Pada Viparita Dandasana*
Time: 20 to 30 seconds
Indications: Stretching; opens chest
Contraindications: Wrist injuries; shoulders injuries; back injuries; neck injuries

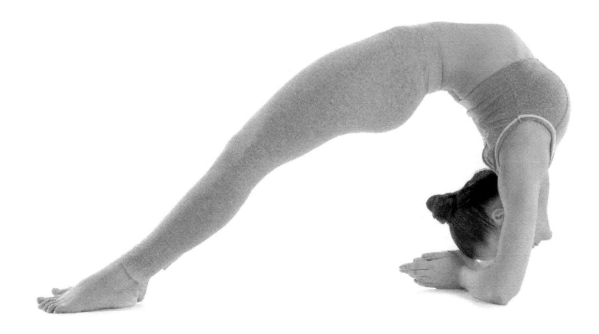

The Upward Facing Two Foot Staff Pose is an expert backbend pose reserved for yogis who have mastered the Upward Bow Pose. It stretches the entire front body, and it strongly puffs the chest.

I recommend rolling up a sticky mat to support your elbows; this will make the pose more comfortable.

To perform this exercise, you must:

1. Prepare for the Upward Bow Pose: Just lie on your back, rest your feet on the floor with your heels under your knees, and step your feet a little more than hip-width.

2. Bend your arms, and then rest your palms, shoulder-width apart, on the floor beside your ears, with your fingertips facing your shoulders.
3. Push your knees away from your torso, and then lift your hips, shoulders, and head off the floor as you extend your arms.
4. Broaden your shoulder blades and drag them toward your tailbone, lifting your shoulders to lighten the load on your arms.
5. Bend your arms and rest the crown of your head on the floor between your hands and feet. Try to keep your elbows shoulder-width apart and directly over your wrists.
6. To avoid compressing your neck, push your hands into the floor and drag your shoulder blades toward your tailbone again. Try to keep your chest lifted.
7. Slide your hands past your ears to cup the back of your head, shifting more weight onto your forearms, and then interlace your fingers behind your head.
8. Push through your inner elbows and wrists to lift your chest, raising your head off the floor. As you tilt your head, push your inner heels down.
9. Your head may seem "glued" to the ground, but that's okay. If you do lift your head, the pose becomes easier. It will allow your upper arms to *directly* support your weight, thus lightening the load on your muscles. Be particularly careful about straining your shoulder joints; don't push them beyond your elbows.
10. Distribute your weight between your elbows and wrists; do this by keeping your elbows shoulder-width apart.
11. If you feel like you can't straighten your legs completely, staying with your head raised and your heels below your knees is fine. However, do try to straighten your legs by walking your feet away until they're almost straight. You will have to plant your feet as you stretch through your calves for the last push.
12. Put the crown of your head back on the floor, inside the cup of your hands. Then press your elbows into the floor and draw your shoulder blades toward your tailbone to help your shoulders stay lifted.
13. Hold the pose for 20 to 30 seconds. To end this pose, you must walk your feet back under your knees, while you remain on your crown. Then you return your palms to the floor next to your ears, making sure your hands are directly below your elbows. Push up with your hands to lift your head, and then tuck your chin and tailbone as you roll your spine back toward the floor.

Tortoise Pose

Focus: Neck; shoulders; arms; legs; spine
Level: Advanced
Sanskrit Name: *Kurmasana*
Time: 30 seconds to 1 minute
Indications: Stretching; strengthening; abdominal stimulation
Contraindications: Knee injuries; back injuries; pregnancy; disk hernias; sciatica

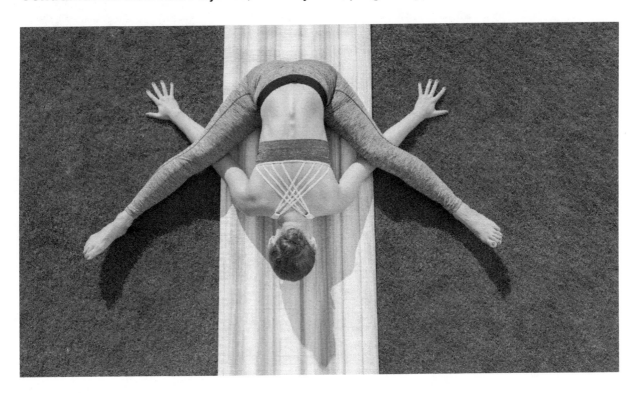

The Tortoise Pose is an advanced pose that requires fine control of your limbs and a lot of strength.

This pose stretches the neck, head, and shoulders; stimulates the abdominal organs; releases tension from the lumbar and sacrum areas of the body; and lengthens the spine.

To perform this exercise, you must:

1. Sit down, keeping your legs spread out in front of you and your back upright. Set your arms alongside your hips and keep your legs shoulder-width apart.
2. Push your thighs into the ground and lift your chest.

3. Bend your knees and bring your feet closer to your hips. Stretch your arms forward, in between your legs, and tilt your torso down along with your arms.
4. Bend your knees even further to let your shoulders go beneath your knees, and then shift your extended arms to the sides.
5. Bring your thighs inward, and then apply pressure through them onto your shoulders to push your chest forward and down. Extend your legs, and try to keep your inner thighs nestled with your side ribs.
6. Bring your head down, chin touching the ground, and gaze down. Extend your arms to the sides as much as possible.
7. Hold the pose for 30 seconds to a minute, breathing easily. Come out gently and slowly by lifting your chest and arms off the ground.

Yoga Sequences

A yoga sequence is the combination of a few poses together in a continuous flow. A good yogi trains with specific sequences. For every need you might have, there's a sequence, although you can always make your own! You will find here ten sequences that are great for beginners and have specific aims. When performing a sequence, take all the time you need, remember to bread properly and do as much as you can without feeling intense pain to avoid injury. We have illustrated the sequence with the images of poses included in this book.

10-Minute Back Pain Sequence

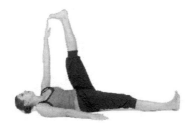 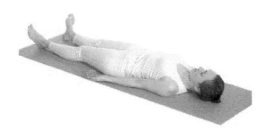

This "lite" yoga sequence offers you 10 minutes' worth of poses to release the tension from your back. Be sure *not to* press your lower back into the floor during this sequence.

1. Lie prone on the ground, belly up, and drag your right knee toward your chest, holding onto your right shin with both hands. Release and switch to the left. Repeat this exercise 4 more times. All in all, you should take at least a minute in this stage.
2. Enter the Reclining Hand to Toe Pose, and hold each side for 30 seconds.
3. Enter the Reclining Hand to Toe Pose, but instead of raising your legs toward the ceiling, stretch them to their respective sides while gazing forward. Loop a strap if you can't reach your feet comfortably. Hold each side for 30 seconds.
4. Enter the Reclining Hand to Toe Pose, but stretch your legs up, and lean them towards the opposite side as much as you can without turning your torso and other leg (i.e., lift your right leg up and lean it to the left). Hold each side for 30 seconds.

217

5. Bring both of your knees toward your chest, rest your right ankle above your left knee, on the left thigh, and hold your left thigh. Hold for a minute and then switch to the other side.
6. Close with the Corpse Pose, holding for 3 minutes.

20-Minute Back Pain Sequence

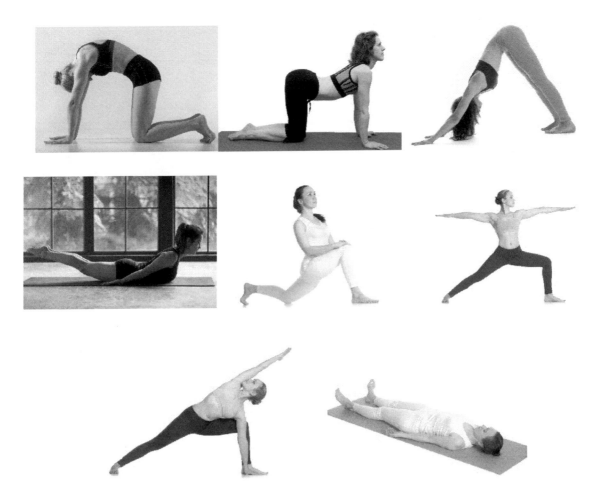

This is a continuation from the past sequence. Instead of closing with the corpse pose, perform this sequence *after* finishing the previous one.

1. Perform a body wave by entering the Cat Pose, then the Cow Pose, and so on, 5 times. Allow 1 breath per stage. It should be around a minute.
2. Perform the Downward Facing Dog Pose. Hold the pose for 6 to 10 breaths, for at least a minute.
3. Enter the Locust Pose. Keep your legs from touching each other if you can, and don't clench your buttocks. Hold the pose for 4 breaths, lower, rest, and repeat another 3 times.
4. Go into the Low Lunge Pose, and hold each side for a minute.
5. Go into the Low Lunge Pose, but raise your back leg into diagonal relative to the ground to enter High Lunge, and rest your hands on your hips. Hold each side for a minute.

6. Go one last time into High Lunge, come into the Warrior Pose II, and then the Extended Side Angle Pose. Hold for a minute, then come back into the High Lunge Pose and perform the exercise again with your legs reversed.
7. Close with 3 minutes of the Corpse Pose.

Ankle Boosting Sequence

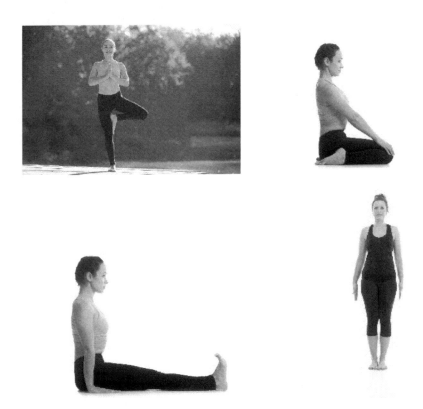

Our ankles carry our weight and allow us to move, and they deserve attention. Unfortunately, not many realize this until it's too late.

This sequence will help you reverse the damage of the past and fortify your ankles against injury and wear for the years to come.

1. Open the sequence with the Tree Pose, but use one leg as a stand and the other as a brace. Hold the pose for 5 to 10 even breaths, and then switch to the other side and repeat.
2. Go into the Hero Pose, but loop a strap around your ankles. Position your ankles so that the balls of your feet are on the ground, and sit on your ankles. Pull the strap taut between your legs. Hold for 5 breaths, and then rest the tops of your feet on the floor. Hold for 5 breaths and then repeat the session one more time.
3. Enter the Staff Pose, ankles pinned together and dorsiflexed, and turn the soles of your feet inward, as if you were saying "Namaste" with your feet. Lastly, reverse the action. Repeat these movements 10 to 20 times to stimulate your ankles.

4. Lastly, part from the Mountain Pose, push your toes into the ground, and then lower to the ground again. Repeat 10 to 20 times. There's no need to rush either motion!

Sun Salutation

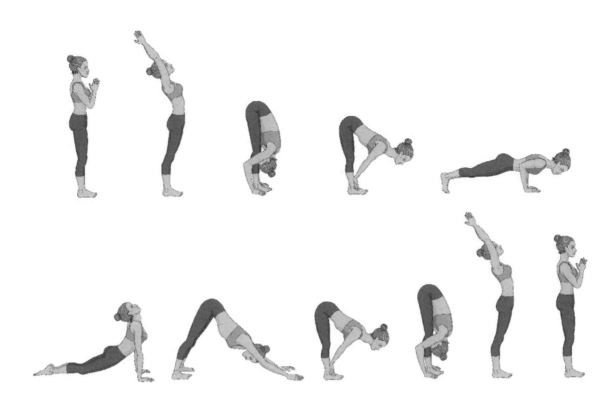

1. Start in Mountain Pose, keeping your palms together as in prayer.
2. Inhale, stretch your arms over your head, and arch your back.
3. Exhale as you bend forward, with your hands reaching for the floor on the outer side of the feet, as in standing forward bend. You may also bend your knees.
4. Inhale as you stretch your right leg backwards. Tuck in your toes so your foot is straight. Exhale.
5. Inhale as you bring the left leg back to place it closer to the right foot. Now your legs will be straight and your body will be in one straight line from back to heels.
6. Exhale and bend your elbows to bring your torso closer to the ground. Your body will be parallel to the floor.
7. Place your chin, chest, knees, and toes on the floor, keeping your hips lifted.
8. Inhale, lift your torso up, and arch your back, straightening your hands. Lift your knees. Now you will be on your palms and the front sides of your feet in Upward Facing Dog Pose.

9. Exhale. Raise your hips high and place your feet on the ground, stretching your arms and legs in Downward Facing Dog Pose.

10. Inhale as you bring your right leg forward to place it on the inner side of your right palm, as in high lunge pose.

11. Exhale, bring your left leg forward, and place the left foot close to the right foot. Stretch your knees and assume standing forward bend.

12. Inhale, lift your torso and your arms over your head and draw the palms down in front of your chest as in prayer.

Standing Yoga Sequence

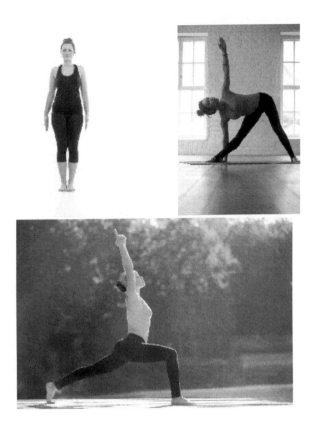

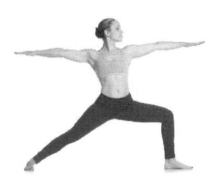

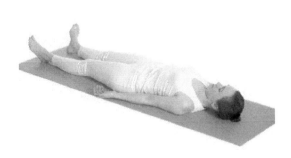

1. Start in Mountain Pose.
2. Inhale and bend backwards, with your arms stretched over your head.
3. Exhale as you come forward, and bend to place your palms on the floor by the sides of your feet, or behind your ankles.
4. Place your legs few feet apart, and stretch your hands sideways. Bend towards your right and place your right palm on the floor, close to your right foot, in Extended Triangle Pose. Repeat the same thing on the other side.
5. From the extended triangle pose, rise and stand straight. Twist your torso to your right and place your right hand on the outer side of the left foot.

6. Turn your right foot towards your right at a 90 degree angle, and your left foot slightly towards your right. Turn your torso to your right, stretch your hands sideways at shoulder-height and over your head. Bend your right knee until the knee is in line with your right ankle. Bring the palms together over your head in Warrior Pose I.

7. From warrior I pose, bring the palms sideways and stretch the arms over the legs. Turn your head forwards, in Warrior Pose II.

8. Release warrior II pose, and bring your feet together and your hands to your sides in mountain pose.

9. Relax in Corpse Pose.

Seated Yoga Sequence

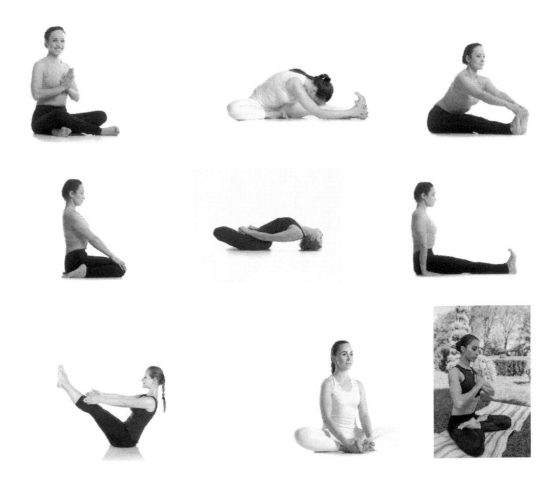

1. Start in Easy Pose, in which you sit on the floor, crossing your legs with your palms on your knees.
2. Stretch your right leg forward, and do Head to Knee Forward Bend Pose.
3. Repeat Head to Knee Forward Bend Pose, extending the left leg.
4. Now, stretch both the legs and perform Seated Forward Bend.
5. Bend your legs to take a kneeling position. Lift your buttocks, bring your big toes together, and sit in the space between the heels. Keep your spine straight and place your palms on your knees.
6. Lift your buttocks, place your legs hip-width apart and sit down in the space, keeping your lower legs close to the outer side of your thighs, in Hero Pose.
7. From hero pose, lean back to perform Reclining Hero Pose.
8. Release your legs and stretch them forward. Place your hands by your sides, keeping your legs at 45 degrees.
9. Lift your legs straight so they are perpendicular to the floor.
10. Place your legs back, get up, and sit in Staff Pose.

11. From staff pose, lift your legs up and balance on the sit bones to perform Boat Pose.
12. Place your legs on the floor, bring the feet together, and perform Bound Angle Pose.
13. Stretch your legs, and place the feet on the opposite thighs. Sit straight, and keep your palms on the knees in chin mudra, for Lotus Pose.

Mind & Body Balance Sequence

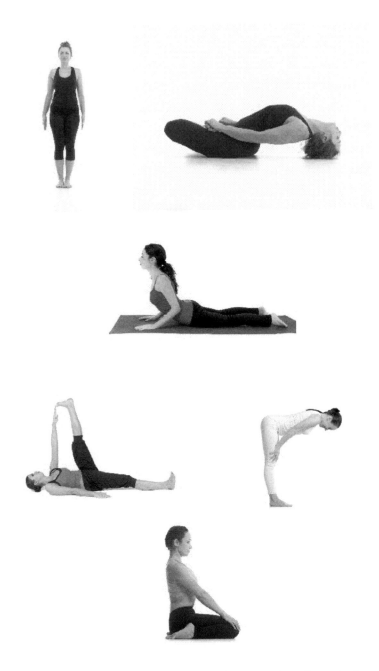

Yoga is more than physical exercise. Some of us tend to forget about this, but we will reconnect with the meditative aspect of yoga in this sequence.

Hold the poses for at least 30 seconds, but keep your breathing even and controlled.

1. Open with the Mountain Pose. Try to hold it for 9 even breaths.

2. Open your chest with the Reclined Hero Pose. Feel free to use a bolster below the fifth thoracic vertebra, and there's no problem with fully extending your legs either.
3. Go into the Cobra Pose.
4. Go into the Reclining Hand to Toe Pose.
5. Go into the Standing Half Forward Bend Pose.
6. Lie supine on a folded blanket and concentrate on your breathing for 10 minutes. Keep your palms up.
7. Enter into a comfortable seated pose (such as the Hero Pose) and meditate. Use one hand to massage your chest, and think of love and gratitude for your life. Hold this meditation for 5 minutes, then release gently and open your eyes, slowly and smiling.

12-Minute Sequence for Bone Health

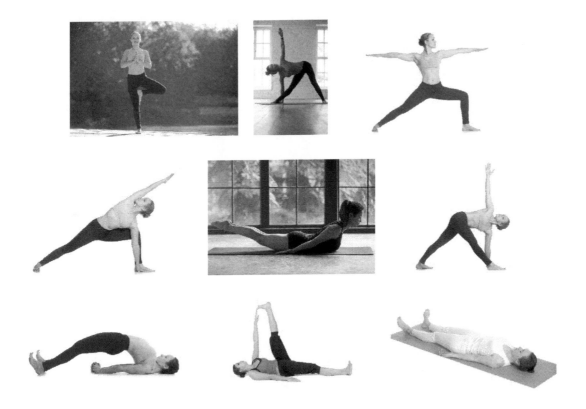

Whether you're interested in staving off osteoporosis or strengthening your bones for the sake of becoming fitter, this 12-minute yoga sequence will boost your protective bone mass.

Try holding each pose for about 30 seconds (per side too, when applicable).

1. Start with the Tree Pose.
2. Go into the Extended Triangle Pose.
3. Go into the Warrior Pose II.
4. Go into the Extended Side Angle Pose.
5. Go into the Locust Pose.
6. Go into the Revolved Triangle Pose.
7. Go into the Bridge Pose.
8. Go into the Reclining Hand to Toe Pose.
9. Go into the Reclining Hand to Toe Pose, but instead of raising your legs toward the ceiling, stretch them out to their respective sides while gazing up.
10. Close with the Corpse Pose.

Mixing yoga exercises with cardio and strength training will yield even better results!

Contentment Cultivation Sequence

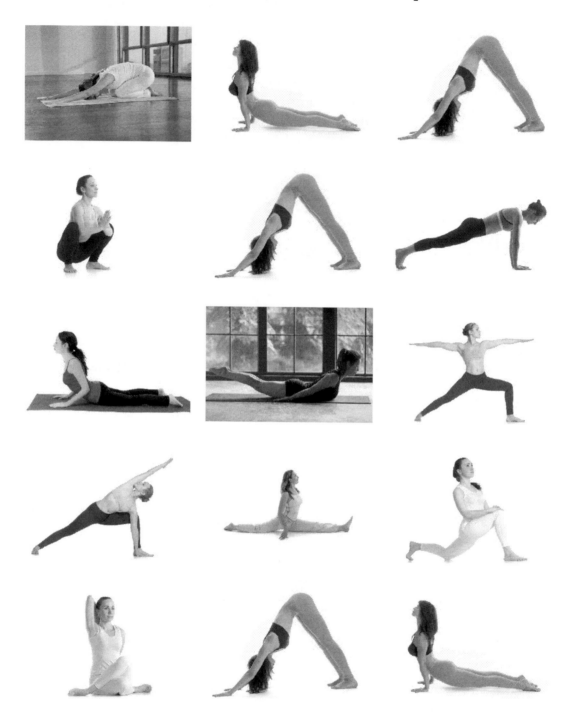

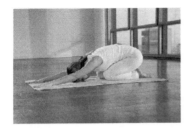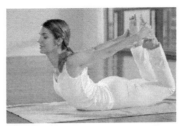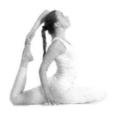
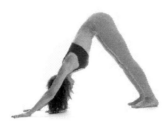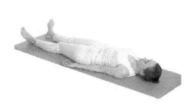

If the waves of life seem unforgiving, there's no need to fret!

Try this sequence to prove to yourself that you have, within your body, the grace and strength needed to navigate through those choppy waters.

Open the sequence with three to five rounds of Sun Salutations, and then carry on with the poses, holding each for at least 30 seconds:

1. Go to the Child Pose, then into the Upward Facing Dog Pose, and lastly the Downward Facing Dog Pose.
2. Go into the Garland Pose.
3. Go into the Downward Facing Dog Pose, but instead of leaving your arms on the ground, grasp each outer ankle with the opposite arm (i.e., grab your right outer ankle with your left hand) for 3 to 5 breaths.
4. Enter the Downward Facing Dog Pose again, but this time, step your right foot in between your hands, move your back foot a few inches to the left, and dig your back heel into the Earth. Reach your arms behind you, toward the ceiling, and interlace your fingers. Hold the position for a few breaths and switch to the other side.
5. Enter the Plank Pose, but walk your hand and lower your torso until you're resting on top of your forearms.
6. Go into the Cobra Pose.
7. Enter the Locust Pose and try clasping your hands together.
8. Go into the Warrior Pose II.
9. Go into the Extended Side Angle Pose.
10. Go into the Monkey Pose, and then rise into the Low Lunge Pose. Once done, reverse your legs and repeat.

11. Enter the Low Lunge and put your arms into the Cow Face Pose.
12. Go into the Downward Facing Dog Pose, then into the Upward Facing Dog Pose (make sure your knees don't reach the floor). Repeat from five to twenty times, and end by resting in the Child Pose.
13. From the Child Pose, rest on your forearms, slide your knees wide open, and turn your feet until your ankles and knees are in line (each ankle forming a 90° angle with your hips).
14. Puff your chest and raise your legs in the Bow Pose.
15. Enter the One-Legged King Pigeon Pose I, but place your hands on the ground beside your front knee, palms off the floor, with your fingertips resting flat on the ground. Lift back and bend forward on one side three to five times, step into the Downward Facing Dog Pose, and then repeat the exercise on the other side.
16. Close the sequence with the Corpse Pose.

Supine Sequence

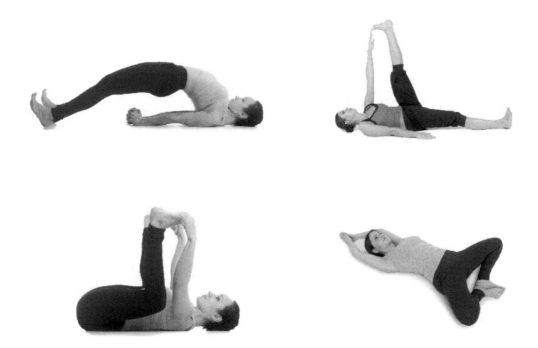

1. Lie down on the floor, stretch your legs out, and place your hands by your sides.
2. Bend your legs and place your feet on the floor, keeping the ankles aligned with your knees vertically. Lift your hips off the floor, and perform Bridge Pose.
3. From bridge pose, lie down on your back. Bend your knees and keep the soles of your feet on the floor. Place the right ankle on the outer side of the left thigh. Pull your left foot toward your body, and slide your right hand through the legs and curl it around the left thigh. You can also clasp your left thigh with your hands. Pressing with your hands, draw the left thigh closer to your chest. Relax your feet.
4. Release the pose, and stretch your legs forward. Relax and twist your torso to your left, placing your right foot outside the left thigh.
5. After that, stretch your legs and keep your hands by your sides. Bend your right leg and draw the right foot towards your chest. Hold the big toe of the right foot with your right hand, and stretch the leg straight in Reclining Hand-to-Toe Pose. Repeat the same with the other leg. Stretch your legs.
6. Bend your legs and bring your knees forward. Hold your feet to go into Happy Baby Pose.

7. Place your legs back on the floor, bring the soles of the feet together, and perform Reclining Bound Angle Pose.

Conclusion

Yoga is more than mere stretching. It exercises the body, mind, and spirit.

It's probably not news to you that yoga is perfect for your wellbeing; the modern popularity of yoga has spread that message very effectively. But now that you've learned so much about yoga and its many benefits, you have a much better idea of the reasons for that.

The truth is that yoga, and the way we practice it through meditation and the asanas, reflects how one should live life.

Think about all the times we try to rush things, desperately trying to achieve our goals in ever smaller amounts of time because the world has become so fast. That's not inherently wrong; in fact, the intentions are good—but good intentions alone don't shape us.

The only thing that can bring you closer to your goals is constant practice, introspection, and patience. Yoga is about all that.

Practicing yoga is about flexing a little bit every day for months just to break the tightness of our body. It's about regulating our breath and mind to endure extreme bodily poses that defy our sense of balance. Lastly, it's about knowing that the best poses will require a considerable time investment.

No matter how much you rush or how hard you press, some things simply require time and repetition. Simple as that.

This is an invaluable message for most of us today. We can't afford to get carried away by the mentality of instant gratification. We're bound to crash into a stone wall of ineptitude sooner or later if we don't start doing things with care and consistency.

I hope this book has given you more than a handful of bodily poses and sequences to train your body; in truth, I hope you realize these core life precepts. They're far more valuable.

That is not to diminish the impacts of yoga on your health. If you're like me, and you work a lot of hours at the computer, you might be accustomed to the stiff feeling of your body. Some days you don't even want to sit at all. That is one perfect reason to start practicing yoga.

With just 20 minutes each day, you can breathe more life and energy into your seemingly spent body. The surge of power will allow you to achieve more, but besides this tangible surge of wellbeing, think about how good would it be to reconnect with your respiration and your thoughts every day.

We've become disconnected from our inner self. In a single span of time we think of *so many* different and unrelated things that we can't even follow our own train of thought.
Yoga *demands* you stop for a moment, forcing you to reflect.

Indeed, yoga is truly a wonderful school of philosophy and exercise. Practicing it, and doing it honestly, with an open mind and an open heart, will net you a multitude of benefits that go far beyond stretching both of your legs parallel to the ground.

Good luck yogi, your ascetic journey has just barely begun!

Made in the USA
Las Vegas, NV
25 August 2023